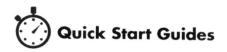

Quick Start Guides

The Essential
HEALTHY GUT
DIET
RECIPE BOOK

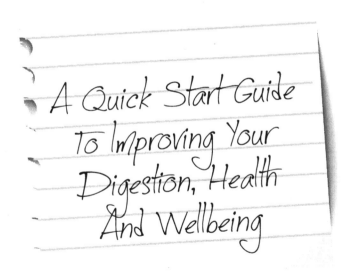

A Quick Start Guide To Improving Your Digestion, Health And Wellbeing

Over 80 Delicious Gut-Friendly Recipes

First published in 2017 by Erin Rose Publishing

Text and illustration copyright © 2017 Erin Rose Publishing

Design: Julie Anson

ISBN: 978-1-911492-12-2

A CIP record for this book is available from the British Library.

DISCLAIMER: This book is for informational purposes only and not intended as a substitute for the medical advice, diagnosis or treatment of a physician or qualified healthcare provider. The reader should consult a physician before undertaking a new health care regime and in all matters relating to his/her health, and particularly with respect to any symptoms that may require diagnosis or medical attention.

While every care has been taken in compiling the recipes for this book we cannot accept responsibility for any problems which arise as a result of preparing one of the recipes. The author and publisher disclaim responsibility for any adverse effects that may arise from the use or application of the recipes in this book. Some of the recipes in this book include nuts and eggs. If you have an egg or nut allergy it's important to avoid these. It is recommended that children, pregnant women, the elderly or anyone who has an immune system disorder avoid eating raw eggs.

CONTENTS

Stage 1 Recipes

Condiments & Dips

Stage 2 Recipes

Breakfast

Lunch

INTRODUCTION

If you have digestive problems, allergies, intolerances, skin conditions and struggle to lose weight, it may be down to an imbalance in your gut bacteria. You'll be pleased to know that with simple dietary changes you can improve your digestion, health and vitality!

Nutritionists have known for years about the effects of yo-yo dieting, sugars, starches and antibiotic overuse and the long term effects such as a 'leaky gut', diabetes and inflammatory diseases. Now you too can learn how to have a healthy gut, like so many people world-wide.

By increasing the diversity and volume of your gut bacteria, you can reap the benefits of a healthier and more efficient digestive system. In this book you can discover your food triggers and learn how to overcome them to end the discomfort and frustration of chronic digestive issues - plus you can lose extra pounds too.

In this **Quick Start Guide**, you will learn which foods to eat and which foods to avoid to optimise your digestion together with lots of useful tips.

This book contains over 80 simple and delicious gut-friendly recipes to boost your immune system and increase your vitality. The aim of this book is to make healthy eating easy, so the tasty, nutritional recipes are clearly laid out for each stage of the 4 week plan.

Once the 4 weeks is up, you can maintain your digestive health and be in the best shape you can be. So if you are ready to improve your wellbeing then this simple 4-week plan is for you!

Are you ready to get started? Let's begin!

Your Key To Great Health

Your digestive system plays an essential role and really is the key to optimal health. It begins with the input of nutrients and the conversion of food to nutrients is a complex and amazing process.

The gut is also referred to as the 2nd brain and the enteric nervous system connects the digestive system and the brain, which communicate through neurons in the guts establishing the mind-gut connection. Metaphorically, we say we can't 'digest' something we've read or heard and likewise our 'gut instinct' is a combination of what is felt and understood by the mind and the stomach. Stress often affects our digestion as chemicals and hormones are released.

The whole process of digestion is aided by some critically important inhabitants of our digestive tract – the microorganisms and bacteria which live there. Your digestive system is literally teeming with life.

The term given to the colonies of microorganisms living within us is the 'microbiome'. These microbes are essential to your hormones, immune system and metabolism. Humans host trillions of bacteria all along our digestive system from start to finish. So, don't be alarmed at the thought of the bacteria in your gut as they work with us.

Our relationship with these bacteria is mutually beneficial in that they require the right conditions in our body in order to reproduce. Let's just look at the difference between harmful and helpful bacteria. It's a complex balance of bacteria which cause good or ill health. The 'gut flora' as it is also known, has colonies of various bacteria. Our gut provides a barrier to pathogens and harmful bacteria and all is well when the balance is harmonious but when good bacteria are in short supply, it weakens the integrity of the gut and increases the risk of disease.

Salmonella, E. coli and campylobacter are examples of harmful bacteria which cause severe illness and they are obviously not what we want in our bodies. On the other side of that microbes like bifidobacterium, lactobacillus, akkermansia, christensenella, butyrate and bacteroidetes we do want in abundance.

So how do we get these good bacteria? Isn't there a pill we can take to provide us with the right balance in the correct amounts? As yet there isn't, and although we can take probiotics as a supplement there is still debate as to how effective they are in reaching along the digestive tract into the small and large intestine, but there is certainly no harm taking probiotics.

So how can we improve our gut bacteria? In the absence of a magic bullet, it requires a change of diet, eliminating foods which promote the growth of harmful bacteria and prevent friendly bacteria from reproducing, then increasing bacterial diversity. That's where you can make a difference. The aim of this diet is to help the good microbes to flourish and improve your digestion, immune system and metabolism. The knock on effect can be reduced inflammation in the body which results in less risk of chronic health conditions like allergies, eczema, IBS and diabetes.

What Is Leaky Gut?

Some of you may be familiar with the term 'leaky gut' which basically describes what happens when your intestines becomes more permeable, allowing food particles to pass through, causing your body to react with inflammation. This inflammation is harmful all round and can also lead to your body storing excess fat.

A healthy gut made up with a great number of diverse bacteria will prevent your gut lining becoming too permeable. Having too many unhelpful bacteria in the gut can lead to sugar cravings and cravings for starchy carbohydrates which particular bacteria like candida can thrive on.

What Harms The Gut?

An Overuse Of Antibiotics

Overuse of antibiotics is a major cause of gut problems due to their effect on the gut flora. Yes, antibiotics can be necessary and life-saving but the overuse of antibiotics for minor issues, viruses and their preventative use can harm the microbial diversity, weakening it, leaving you vulnerable to recurrent infections. Antibiotics inhibit the growth of bacteria (good and bad) and a study by The University of Valencia showed that after a course of antibiotics the gut was less able to digest certain foods, particularly iron. Research also shows that babies born by caesarean have less diverse gut bacteria, possibly due to the mother being given antibiotics preventively before birth. Breastfeeding is a natural way of ensuring better health for infants.

The repeated overuse of antibiotics is considered to be a major factor in gut dysfunction caused by poor bacteria, leading to increased intestinal permeability (leaky gut) causing inflammation and allergies due to certain micro particles leaking from the gut.

The good news is that gut bacteria can be improved with a healthy diet of plenty of fresh vegetables, fruit, quality protein and the assistance of pre and probiotics.

Sugar

Sugar is found more commonly in everyday food than you may think and is added to even savoury processed foods, marinades, sauces and relishes. Aside from being linked with diabetes, cancer, heart disease and many other illnesses it is detrimental to the gut bacteria. Sugar encourages the growth of harmful bacteria such as fungus and parasites which produce toxins. So as well as avoiding adding cakes, sweets and biscuits, look out for the hidden sugars in your diet and read the labels of all foods. It may not be listed as 'sugar' so look out for it by another name and check out the list.

- Agave syrup
- Barley Malt
- Beet sugar
- Cane juice crystals
- Carob syrup
- Coconut sugar
- Corn syrup and high fructose corn syrup
- Date sugar
- Dehydrated fruit juice
- Dextrin
- Dextrose
- Ethyl maltol
- Fructose and fructose syrup
- Fruit juice concentrate
- Glucose syrup
- Golden syrup
- Invert sugar syrup
- Sucrose
- Maltose
- Malt syrup
- Maltodextrin
- Maple syrup
- Molasses
- Palm sugar
- Rice syrup
- Refiners syrup
- Treacle

Artificial Sweeteners

Research has shown that artificial sweeteners such as those used in sugar-free soft drinks, sweets and processed foods, alter the gut bacteria, changes the metabolism and increases the risk of diabetes. Avoiding sugar is essential to gut health but substituting it with artificial sweeteners may also harm your health. Also studies show that it's not just sugar that causes cravings but sweet tasting foods, like those with added sweeteners, stimulate the brain to crave more. Not what you wanted to hear if you've got a sweet tooth but your taste buds will adjust with your improved diet. If you really need a sugar substitute then try stevia as numerous studies worldwide have found it to be a safe alternative.

Stress

Stress can have a negative effect on digestion due to the effect of cortisol from the adrenals influencing gastric motility, low stomach acid, blood flow and even bacteria. Nervousness and anxiety can often be felt in the gut often with uncomfortable sensations as you respond to a 'gut feeling'. Avoiding stress completely may not be possible but try to take time out for exercise, especially yoga, or meditation or even a peaceful walk. There are countless meditations and mindfulness options on YouTube which can really help you tune out and reset your brain.

Tying in with the stress aspect, caffeine and alcohol can be stimulating and cause inflammation which is why these items are on the 'foods to avoid' list. Some people process both of these much more effectively than others and it is only temporary for the elimination part of the diet although you may want to continue on avoiding it or indulging occasionally. There is yet more good news for red wine. Not only is it a 'sirt' food, (foods which contain the sirtuin activating compound or 'skinny gene') as it contains resveratrol but it contains polyphenols which are abundant in antioxidants, so if you are having a tipple, make it red wine.

Medications

Some medications to treat acid reflux and stomach acid can be detrimental to the digestive flora but that is by no means a recommendation to stop your medication. Always consult your GP before embarking on any changes you wish to make to ensure it's safe for you to do so.

Processed Foods

Processed food which contains little or no fibre from fresh vegetables and fruit will not help your gut health. Also convenience foods often have sugar, sweeteners, gluten and additives in them so they can be preventing the growth of the good guys. A diet which contains too few fresh vegetables and fruits will decrease the diversity of your gut bacteria as fruit and vegetables have a prebiotic effect and encourage the growth of good bacteria.

Fat

A diet high in unhealthy fats can harm your gut. Avoid all foods containing hydrogenated trans fats such as margarines, ready meals, desserts, cakes and biscuits and reading the label you will be able to identify those. Eating healthy fats and oils is great for your health so olive oil, coconut oil and avocados are all still on the menu.

How To Heal Your Gut

Stage 1 – Elimination

- Start by eliminating or reducing all the foods on the 'avoid' list and if this seems overwhelming just remember this is temporary. You can gradually begin to reduce these foods if you like for a few days before beginning the 2 week elimination stage. The aim is to remove from your diet all foods which can irritate the gut and reduce beneficial intestinal bacteria. You are removing foods which prevent your gut from being the best it can be. It will allow you to repair your gut lining and to fully assimilate nutrients from your food effectively, boost your immunity, reduce dysfunction and improve your digestion – just keep your mind on the goal and move forward.

- Some of you may already have coeliac disease or gluten and/or dairy intolerance and have already removed these from your diet – let's remember that is essential in coeliac disease. But even if you aren't aware that certain foods are an issue for you, removing them will allow you to detect what triggers your symptoms. Once you removed the foods on the avoid list you may notice a significant change very quickly, but for others the improvements can take longer.

- Stick to the elimination stage of the diet for 2 weeks, even if you are feeling better and are tempted to start reintroducing foods. It's worth staying on the elimination stage for 2 weeks to give your digestion a well-earned rest and to heal your gut. If you need longer, or your symptoms aren't settling, check that you aren't inadvertently eating an item containing hidden gluten, dairy or sugar. And remember, as always, if your symptoms persist or worsen, always seek your doctor's advice.

Stage 2 – Reintroduction

If you have eliminated the foods to avoid and haven't seen any improvement, you need to speak to your doctor or a qualified nutritionist. Never ignore symptoms of digestive dysfunction and they must always be investigated. A majority of people will see improvements, so where do you go from here?

- Once you've seen a steady and sustained improvement in your symptoms, you can carefully and systematically over the next 2 weeks reintroduce a small portion of other foods starting with those which promote healthy intestinal bacteria; yogurt, kefir, and good quality blue cheese like stilton or Roquefort.

- Only introduce one new food at a time. Allow 2-3 days to make sure you have no reaction before reintroducing another food. It can be tempting to rush into eating new things when your digestion has improved but pace yourself.

- You can also try increasing the portion size, or move on to another food, for instance if you tolerate dairy you could try pulses or vice versa. Try the foods which are good for your gut bacteria first, like live yogurt, before less beneficial dairy foods.

- If you do get a flare up of symptoms from a reintroduced food, revert to eliminating that food until your symptoms disappear and testing another food.

- Your tolerance can change with the health of your gut. Aim to have as wide a variety of healthy foods in your diet as possible and load up those fresh vegetables. Fruit is helpful too but stick to no more than 2 pieces of fruit a day to keep your fruit sugar consumption low.

- While eliminating and reintroducing foods it is very useful to keep a food diary and list any reactions you may have to foods. You can monitor your other details like bowel habits, digestion, weight and energy levels. It's easy to forget what you've eaten and a diary can show you your unique patterns.

- If you have known food allergies, anaphylaxis or are coeliac, it's important to continue to avoid the foods which cause it. If you have a food intolerance eliminating that food may allow you to eat a certain portion of that food without a problem. However this isn't the case if you are coeliac as it's vital to continue being completely gluten-free.

Foods To Avoid

- Sugar including soft drinks, fruit juices, desserts, dried fruit, cakes, cookies, muesli bars, sweets, candy and chocolate bars including those with artificial sweeteners and agave syrup.

- Gluten and starchy carbohydrates such as pasta, white rice, bread, biscuits, crackers, cereals and granola.

- All whole grains including brown rice, wheat, quinoa, barley, oats, and rye. (These can be reintroduced later.)

- Pulses including, cannellini beans, kidney beans, lima beans, barlotti beans, chickpeas (garbanzo beans) and haricot beans.

- Avoid all dairy produce such as milk, cheese, butter, cream, crème fraîche, cream cheeses and yogurt (live yogurt and some cheese can be added at the re-introduction stage).

- Caffeine

- Alcohol

- Nuts and seeds including nut milks and nut butters like peanut butter, almond and cashew nut butter.

Foods You Can Eat

- All meat, including beef, pork, venison, chicken, turkey, duck, goose and seafood, especially oily fish such as salmon, mackerel and sardines.

- Eggs

- Nuts and seeds including, brazil nuts, almonds, walnuts, hazelnuts, peanuts, pecans, pumpkin seeds, sunflower seeds, pine nuts, sesame seeds, flaxseeds (linseeds), chia seeds and nut butters.

- Dairy alternatives, like coconut milk, almond milk, cashew milk and hemp milk, coconut butter and coconut cream.

Vegetables

- Aubergine (eggplant)
- Broccoli
- Courgette (zucchini)
- Cauliflower
- Radish
- Beetroot
- Celeriac
- Swede
- Green Beans
- Kale
- Cabbage

- Beansprouts
- Water chestnuts
- Peas
- Peppers (bell peppers)
- Fennel
- Squash
- Sweet Potatoes
- Avocados
- Olives
- Carrots
- Celery
- Tomatoes
- Spinach
- Lettuce
- Chicory
- Cucumber
- Mange tout
- Sea weeds like nori, kelp and dulse
- Onions
- Garlic
- Leeks
- Asparagus
- Artichoke
- Pak choy (bok choi)
- Pumpkin

- Fresh herbs and spices and condiments such as; ginger, garam masala, curry, cardamom, turmeric, mustard, cumin, pepper, chilli, basil, thyme, coriander (cilantro), chives, oregano, dill, sage, lemon balm and mint.

- Tamari
- Honey
- Apple cider vinegar
- Herb and fruit teas, water and coconut water
- Cacao nibs/ cocoa

Fruit
- Apples
- Pears
- Bananas
- Strawberries
- Pineapple
- Oranges
- Tangerines
- Lychee
- Redcurrants
- Cranberries
- Raspberries
- Blueberries
- Blackberries

- Cherries
- Kiwi Fruit
- Melon
- Grapes
- Mango
- Papaya
- Lemons
- Limes
- Melon
- Oranges
- Tangerines
- Papaya
- Peaches
- Pears
- Pineapple
- Pomegranate
- Redcurrants
- Strawberries

Avoid eating too much fruit as it can have a high fructose (fruit sugar) content, especially very ripe fruit.

Top Tips For Good Gut Health

The following foods can be really beneficial to your gut bacteria so once you have completed the elimination stage you can gradually introduce them. It's a good idea to introduce these before other foods as they boost your gut bacteria diversity really well.

Butter

Butter has had bad press in the past but it's a more natural and healthier alternative to many oil based spreads. Butter is a rich source of energy and butyric acid which is a short-chain fatty acid which can help reduce gut inflammation and aid repair, it curbs hunger and helps balance the metabolism.

Live Yogurt

Live yogurt is considered a superfood by some. The living cultures in yogurt, such as lactobacillus, give your gut bacteria a welcome boost and help your immune system, of which 70% is in the digestive system. The bacteria in yogurt have been found to reach the end of the digestive tract which means they have survived their journey right through the intestines – the great news is that their benefits reach all corners of your digestive system. It's believed that fat in dairy products can protect and help the transit of the bacteria so always use full-fat yogurt.

Kimchi

It may be an acquired taste but this Korean traditionally made from cabbage, radish and other vegetables and seasoned with spices is a great fermented food containing gut-friendly cultures. You may find it in specialised food shops or you could try making your own.

Sauerkraut

This raw fermented cabbage is commonly eaten in Poland and Germany and isn't widely available in the shops so making your own is the best way forward. It may not seem appealing but this cultured vegetable is loaded with lactobacillus which improves the flora of the digestive tract and helps digestion. We've included a sauerkraut recipe in this book so you can have a go. It contains more good bacteria than live yogurt so well worth adding to your diet.

Blue Cheese

Blue cheeses like, stilton, gorgonzola and Roquefort are excellent probiotics adding bacteria diversity to the gut. They contain active live cultures which benefit the digestive system. Do eat them in moderation and in small quantities as they do contain a lot of fat.

Kefir

This is a fermented dairy drink and great probiotic. It's produced by adding cultures known as kefir 'grains' to milk and letting it multiply for at least 24 hours. Kefir tastes similar to yogurt and much of the lactose is turned into lactic acid so can be tolerated better by those who are lactose intolerant.

Pistachio Nuts

Pistachios contain polyphenols and fibre and are great butyrate bacteria promoting food so they are a welcome addition to your diet.

Resistant Starch

Just like it sounds, resistant starch is a type of fibre which remains almost intact until it reaches the colon at the end of the digestive tract where it sweeps away toxins and harmful bacteria and feeds the beneficial bacteria. Resistant starch is found in potatoes which are cooked then cooled. This makes potatoes great for a healthy gut.

Intermittent Fasting

If you've missed the hype and praise for intermittent fasting, this is basically where you restrict food intake and calories for a certain period of time. It can be 2 days a week as in the 5:2 diet or you can restrict food intake for 12-14 hours overnight. The upshot of fasting is it's not just a successful weight loss tool but it allows certain healthy bacteria which are responsible for weight loss, to increase in the gut when there is no food available, allowing this particular strain to thrive. It's also so easy to do. Eating in the early evening and having your last meal of the day then will allow an extended time overnight when you're digestive system can rest and in particular those amazing 'skinny' bacteria which helps protect the gut lining and reduces inflammation when there is no food in the way.

Avoid over-eating which can hamper your digestive system. Keep to regular meal times and try to avoid snacking in between.

As you know digestion begins in the mouth, so chew your food well and eat slowly. It will let your gut know food is on its way and kick start the production of digestive enzymes.

IBS & the FODMAPS

The FODMAP diet has been a tried and tested and is a very effective diet for sufferers of severe IBS and has been endorsed by doctors and patients alike.

FODMAP is an abbreviation for **F**ermentable **O**ligosaccharides, **D**isaccharides, **M**onosaccharides and **P**olyols which have been found to be common triggers found in everyday foods and can cause digestive problems.

FODMAP's are carbohydrates found in everyday foods and in some cases otherwise healthy foods, such as apples, garlic and onions which your digestive system can struggle to break down, causing pain, bloating, constipation and diarrhoea.

Often once these foods are removed the symptoms can disappear. Following the healthy gut diet can benefit most people and we mention the FODMAP diet here because if your symptoms are severe you might benefit from removing some or all FODMAP foods from your diet, at least temporarily until improvement has been achieved.

The low FODMAP diet was researched and developed by an Australian team, Dr Sue Shepherd and Dr Peter Gibson at Monash University in Melbourne, who discovered that a diet low in FODMAP foods which contain certain sugars can help resolve stubborn and severe IBS. We mention it in this book as something to consider if your digestion is really out of balance and it may be worth looking into the FODMAP diet which similarly involves elimination and reintroduction of possible food triggers. Ultimately, it's working out what works for you.

Getting Started

Depending on the severity of your symptoms you can either get started straight away on the elimination stage or gradually ease yourself into it. If you usually experience a lot of wind or cramping you may feel more comfortable doing things gradually and gently. It is best to start to reduce/ eliminate sugar and processed foods straight away to start your recovery. Let your symptoms and lifestyle guide you as to what is best.

If you have an event coming up such as a party you may wish to start your gut diet after it. Generally, the sooner the better so you can experience the benefits.

To begin with, go through your kitchen cupboards, reading the labels of foods to identify where the pitfalls lie. For instance look out for sugar, wheat and dairy which has been added to everyday foods.

Stock you fridge with fresh foods and make it easy to meal plan. Familiarise yourself with the foods you can eat so that you are organised and can lay your hands on something quick, simple and tasty to eat which will prevent you from being tempted by ready-made foods or unhealthy snacks.

Check out the recipes and aim to make something which appeals to you. That way you can look forward to something you know you'll enjoy, particularly in the early stages so you can avoid feeling deprived.

In recipes which require the use of stock (broth) you can use bone broth, the recipe for which is on page 68. If you make a large batch and store some in the freezer you can have some ready to add, saving you time and energy.

Making more than you need for one meal so you can store or freeze a portion will save you time in the long run.

For the first 2 weeks, only select recipes from the Stage 1 section then when you begin the Stage 2 on week 3, you can add in helpful foods like honey, yogurt and butter. The Stage 2 recipes contain these but are otherwise free from other foods on your avoid list such as wheat and sugar.

We hope you enjoy the recipes!

Wishing you great health!

Stage 1 Recipes

BREAKFAST

Strawberry & Coconut Smoothie

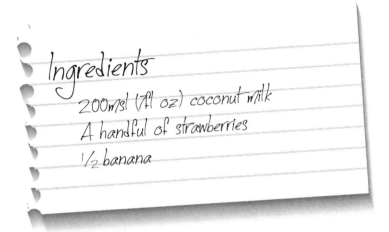

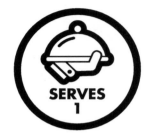

SERVES 1

Ingredients
200msl (7fl oz) coconut milk
A handful of strawberries
½ banana

Method

Toss all the ingredients into a blender and blitz. Pour and enjoy!

Blackberry & Carrot Smoothie

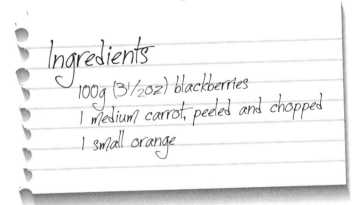

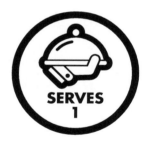

SERVES 1

Ingredients
100g (3½oz) blackberries
1 medium carrot, peeled and chopped
1 small orange

Method

Place all the ingredients into a blender with enough water to cover them and process until smooth. Serve and drink straight away.

Lemon Salad Smoothie

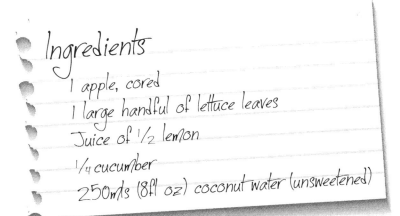

Ingredients

1 apple, cored
1 large handful of lettuce leaves
Juice of ½ lemon
¼ cucumber
250mls (8fl oz) coconut water (unsweetened)

SERVES 1

Method

Place all of the ingredients into a blender and blitz until smooth. Serve straight away.

Minty Green Smoothie

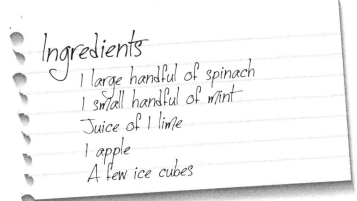

Ingredients

1 large handful of spinach
1 small handful of mint
Juice of 1 lime
1 apple
A few ice cubes

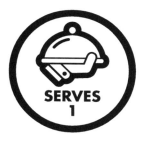

SERVES 1

Method

Place all of the ingredients into a blender and process until smooth. If your blender can't process ice cubes just add them to the glass. Drink straight away.

Creamy Raspberry Smoothie

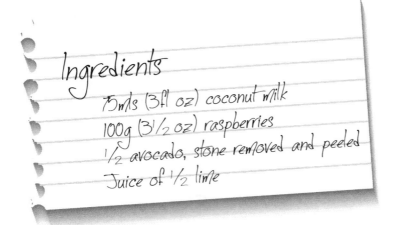

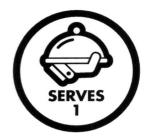
SERVES 1

Ingredients
- 75mls (3fl oz) coconut milk
- 100g (3½ oz) raspberries
- ½ avocado, stone removed and peeled
- Juice of ½ lime

Method

Toss all of the ingredients into a blender. Blitz until smooth and creamy. If it seems too thick you can add some water. Pour and enjoy!

Kiwi Salad Smoothie

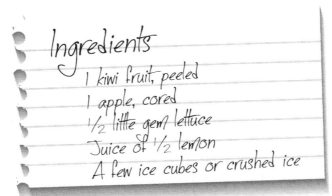

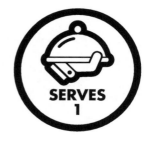
SERVES 1

Ingredients
- 1 kiwi fruit, peeled
- 1 apple, cored
- ½ little gem lettuce
- Juice of ½ lemon
- A few ice cubes or crushed ice

Method

Place all of the ingredients into a food processor with just enough water to cover them. Blitz until smooth. If your blender can't process ice cubes just add them to the glass. Drink straight away.

Pear & Celery Salad Smoothie

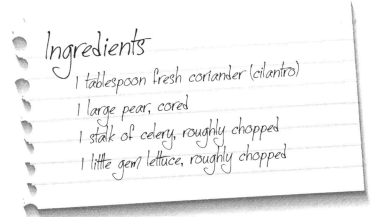

Ingredients

1 tablespoon fresh coriander (cilantro)

1 large pear, cored

1 stalk of celery, roughly chopped

1 little gem lettuce, roughly chopped

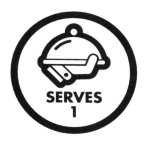

SERVES
1

Method

Place all of the ingredients into a blender with sufficient water to cover them and blitz until smooth.

Green Apple & Pistachio Smoothie

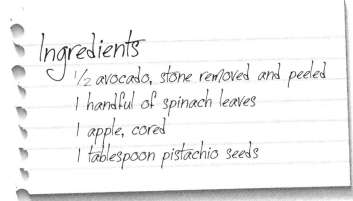

Ingredients

½ avocado, stone removed and peeled

1 handful of spinach leaves

1 apple, cored

1 tablespoon pistachio seeds

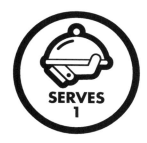

SERVES
1

Method

Put all the ingredients into a blender with just enough water to cover the ingredients. Blitz until smooth. You can add lemon juice for extra zing.

Spinach & Apple Smoothie

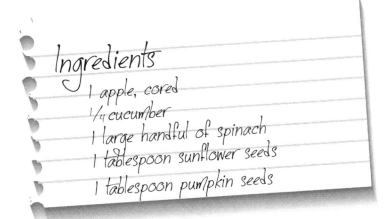

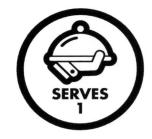

SERVES 1

Method

Place all the ingredients into a blender and add just enough water to cover the ingredients.

Pink Grapefruit & Carrot Zinger

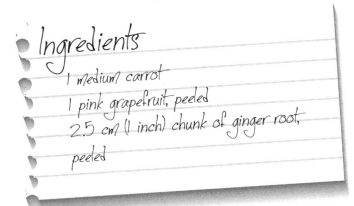

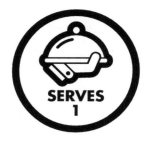

SERVES 1

Method

Place all of the ingredients into a blender with enough water to cover them. Blitz until smooth. Serve and drink straight away.

Basil Blackcurrant Refresher

Ingredients

100g (3½ oz) blackcurrants
4 fresh basil leaves
1 banana
200mls (7fl oz) cold water
Juice of 1 lime

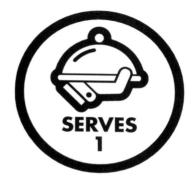

SERVES 1

Method

Place all of the ingredients into a blender and process until smooth. Drink straight away or keep it in the fridge and take little 'shots' throughout the day.

Raspberry Pancakes

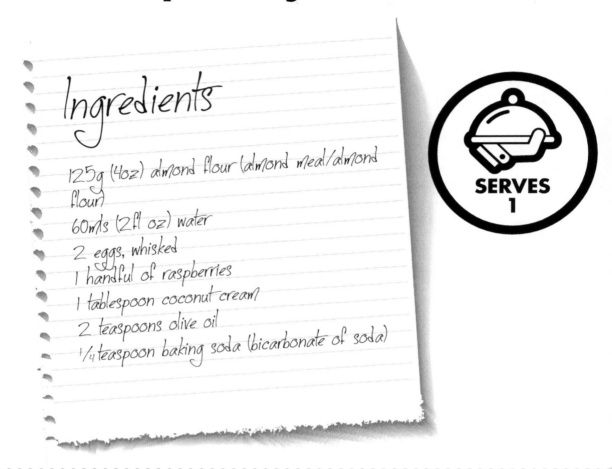

Ingredients

125g (4oz) almond flour (almond meal/almond flour)
60mls (2fl oz) water
2 eggs, whisked
1 handful of raspberries
1 tablespoon coconut cream
2 teaspoons olive oil
1/4 teaspoon baking soda (bicarbonate of soda)

SERVES 1

Method

In a bowl, combine the ground almonds (almond meal/almond flour), eggs and baking powder (bicarbonate of soda) in a bowl and beat the mixture until it is creamy. Heat the oil in a frying pan. Spoon the mixture into the hot pan and as it begins to set pop some raspberries into the pancake. You can make one large one or 2-3 small ones. One the pancakes are golden on one side flip it over to continue cooking. Serve onto a plate with a dollop of coconut cream.

Chocolate & Nut Protein Muesli

Ingredients

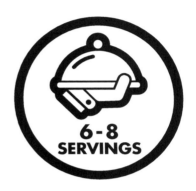

6-8 SERVINGS

200g (7oz) desiccated (shredded) coconut
75g (3oz) chopped cashew nuts
75g (3oz) chopped almonds
75g (3oz) unsalted pistachio nuts, shelled
50g (2oz) chopped hazelnuts
25g (1oz) pumpkin seeds
25g (1oz) cacao nibs or unsweetened chocolate chips
2 tablespoons chia seeds
2 tablespoons 100% cocoa powder
1 teaspoon ground cinnamon

Method

Place all of the ingredients into a large bowl and mix well. Store the muesli in an airtight container until you're ready to use it. Serve with some fresh fruit and some live yogurt.

LUNCH

Root Vegetable Soup

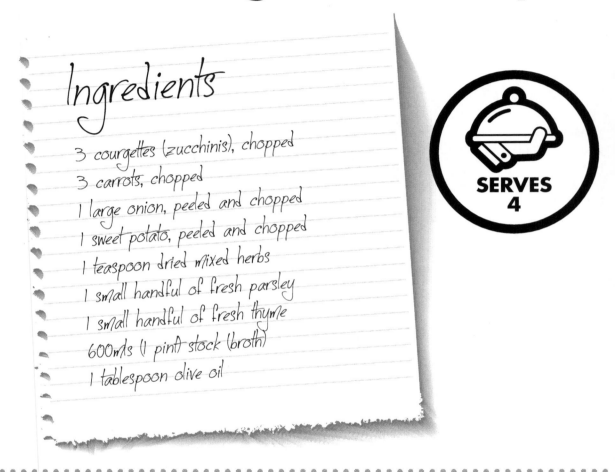

Ingredients

- 3 courgettes (zucchinis), chopped
- 3 carrots, chopped
- 1 large onion, peeled and chopped
- 1 sweet potato, peeled and chopped
- 1 teaspoon dried mixed herbs
- 1 small handful of fresh parsley
- 1 small handful of fresh thyme
- 600mls (1 pint) stock (broth)
- 1 tablespoon olive oil

SERVES 4

Method

Heat the olive oil in a saucepan, add the vegetables and cook for 5 minutes or until they have started to soften. Add the stock (broth) and dried herbs and cook on a medium heat for 20-30 minutes or until the vegetables are cooked through. Stir in the fresh herbs. Use a hand blender or food processor and blitz until smooth. Season and serve.

Gazpacho Soup

Ingredients

5 tomatoes, de-seeded and chopped

1 red pepper (bell pepper), de-seeded and chopped

2 cloves of garlic, chopped

1 cucumber, peeled and chopped

½ teaspoon chilli flakes

2 teaspoons olive oil

2 tablespoons apple cider vinegar

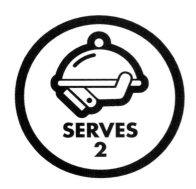

SERVES 2

Method

Place all of the ingredients into a blender and process until smooth and creamy. If it seems too thick you can add a little extra oil or vinegar if you need to. Chill the soup in the fridge for an hour before serving.

Slow Cooked Chicken Broth

SERVES 4

Ingredients

450g (1lb) chicken breasts, chopped

400g (14oz) tinned tomatoes

75g (3oz) cabbage, finely chopped

4 celery stalks, chopped

3 cloves of garlic, chopped

1 onion, peeled and chopped

1 carrot, peeled and diced

1 leek, finely chopped

2 teaspoons dried mixed herbs

1 teaspoon dried coriander (cilantro)

2 tablespoons tomato purée (paste)

1 handful of fresh parsley, chopped

1200mls (2 pints) chicken stock (broth)

300mls (½ pint) hot water

Sea salt

Freshly ground black pepper

Method

Place all of the ingredients into a slow cooker and mix them well. Cook on high for 4- 6 hours. If you prefer your soup thinner you can add a little extra hot water. Serve and enjoy.

Asparagus Soup

Ingredients

450g (14oz) asparagus spears,
2 cloves of garlic, chopped
1/2 courgette (zucchini), chopped
750mls (1 1/2 pints) vegetable stock (broth)
1 tablespoon olive oil

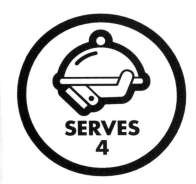

SERVES
4

Method

Heat the oil in a saucepan, add the asparagus, courgette (zucchini) and garlic and cook for 4 minutes. Add in the stock (broth) and cook for 10 minutes. Using a food processor or a hand blender, process the soup until smooth. Serve and enjoy.

Red Pepper, Tomato & Basil Soup

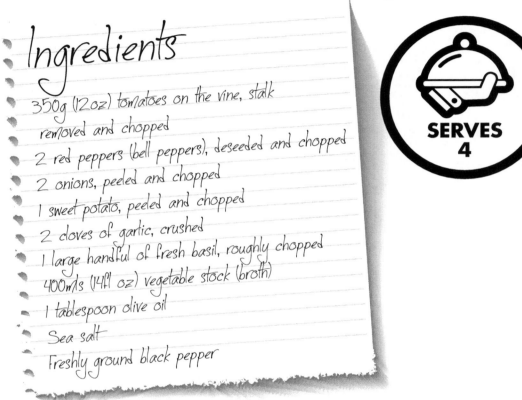

SERVES 4

Ingredients

- 350g (12oz) tomatoes on the vine, stalk removed and chopped
- 2 red peppers (bell peppers), deseeded and chopped
- 2 onions, peeled and chopped
- 1 sweet potato, peeled and chopped
- 2 cloves of garlic, crushed
- 1 large handful of fresh basil, roughly chopped
- 400mls (14fl oz) vegetable stock (broth)
- 1 tablespoon olive oil
- Sea salt
- Freshly ground black pepper

Method

Heat the olive oil in a saucepan, add the onions and cook until they have softened. Add in the sweet potato, tomatoes, red peppers (bell peppers) and garlic and cook for 5 minutes, stirring frequently. Pour in the hot stock (broth) and cook for around 30 minutes and until all the ingredients are cooked through. Stir in half of the basil. Using a hand blender, blitz the soup until smooth. Season with salt and pepper and add in the remaining basil. Serve into bowls and enjoy.

Butternut Squash Soup

Ingredients

- 1 large butternut squash, peeled and de-seeded
- 1 tablespoon olive oil
- 1 large onion, peeled and chopped
- 1 clove of garlic
- 1/4 teaspoon nutmeg
- 1/4 teaspoon ground ginger
- 1/4 teaspoon cinnamon
- 600mls (1 pint) vegetable or chicken stock (broth)
- Sea salt
- Freshly ground black pepper

SERVES 6

Method

Heat the oil in a saucepan, add the onion and garlic and cook until softened. Add in the squash and spices and cook for 3-4 minutes. Pour in the stock (broth) and cook on a low heat for 20 minutes or until the squash is completely cooked. Season with salt and pepper. Using a hand blender or food processor, blitz the soup until smooth.

Coriander, Prawn & Orange Salad

SERVES 2

Ingredients

250g (9 oz) cooked and peeled prawns (shrimps)

50g (2oz) olives

2 tomatoes, chopped

2 tablespoons apple cider vinegar

2 tablespoons extra-virgin olive oil

2 tablespoons fresh coriander (cilantro), chopped

2 little gem lettuce, chopped

1 orange, peeled and chopped

1 red onion, chopped

1 clove of garlic, chopped

1/4 cucumber, peeled and chopped

1/4 teaspoon paprika

Sea salt

Freshly ground black pepper

Method

In a small bowl, combine the oil, vinegar, coriander (cilantro), garlic, paprika, salt and pepper. Add the prawns (shrimps), cucumber, tomatoes, olives and onion and toss them in the dressing. Scatter the lettuce and orange pieces onto a plate. Spoon the prawn mixture over the top. Enjoy!

Seed Crackers

Ingredients

- 75g (3oz) sunflower seeds
- 75g (3oz) chia seeds
- 50g (2oz) ground almonds (almond meal/ almond flour)
- 2 teaspoons herbs de Provence or mixed herbs
- 1 clove of garlic, crushed
- 1/2 teaspoon sea salt
- 250mls (8fl oz) cold water

MAKES 18

Method

In a bowl, combine the sunflower seeds, chia seeds, almonds, garlic, herbs and salt. Pour in the water and mix really well until the ingredients thicken. Grease and line a baking tray and spoon the mixture into it, spreading and smoothing it out. Transfer it to the oven, preheated to 170C/325F and cook for 25 minutes. Remove it and carefully cut it into slices. Return it to the oven and cook for another 25 minutes. Once cooled, store in an airtight container. Use as a snack or serve with salads and dips.

Courgette 'Spaghetti'

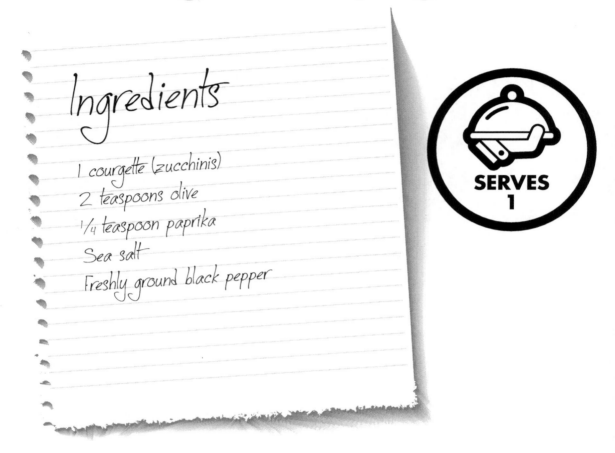

Ingredients

1 courgette (zucchinis)
2 teaspoons olive
1/4 teaspoon paprika
Sea salt
Freshly ground black pepper

SERVES 1

Method

Using a spiraliser, cut the courgette (zucchini) into spirals or if you don't have one simply using a vegetable peeler and cut strips around 1cm (1/2 inch) thick. Place the oil and paprika into a bowl and coat the courgette strips in the oil. Season with salt and pepper. Heat a frying pan and add the strips. Cook for between 2 and 4 minutes, stirring occasionally. Use courgette as an alternative to pasta, rice, potatoes or bread. Although this recipe is for a single portion, simply multiply it using approx. 1 courgette per person.

Vegetables & Aubergine Dip

Ingredients

FOR THE DIP:
1 aubergine (eggplant), chopped
3 tablespoons toasted sesame seeds
1 red chilli
1 teaspoon paprika powder
1 teaspoons olive oil
Juice of 1 lime

FOR THE VEGETABLE CRUDITÉS:
3 carrots, cut into batons
6 sticks of celery, cut into batons
4 spring onions
1 red pepper (bell pepper)
1/4 cucumber, cut into batons
1 small iceberg or romaine lettuce, cut into slices

SERVES ?

Method

Place the aubergine (eggplant) into a steamer and cook until soft. Allow it to cool then place it into a food processor. Add in the sesame seeds, olive oil, chilli, paprika and lime juice. Blitz the mixture in the food processor until smooth. Arrange the vegetables onto a serving plate. Spoon the aubergine dip into a bowl and serve with the vegetables.

Lime & Coriander 'Rice'

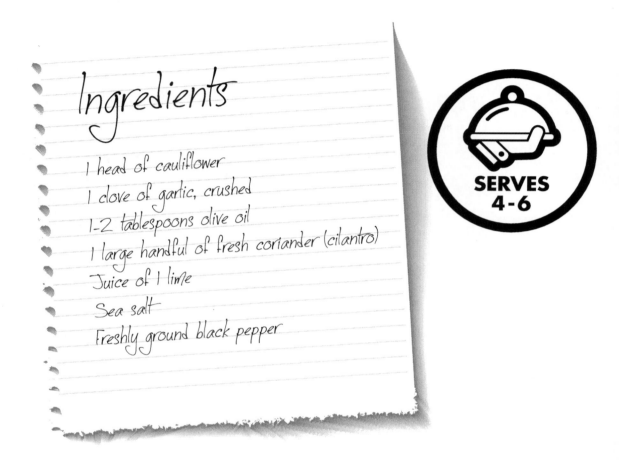

Ingredients

1 head of cauliflower
1 clove of garlic, crushed
1-2 tablespoons olive oil
1 large handful of fresh coriander (cilantro)
Juice of 1 lime
Sea salt
Freshly ground black pepper

SERVES 4-6

Method

Place the cauliflower into a food processor and chop until fine grains. Heat the oil in a frying pan. Stir in garlic and cauliflower and cook for around 6 minutes or until the cauliflower grains are soft. Season with salt and pepper. Add in the lime juice and coriander (cilantro) and mix well. Once it's cooked stir it throughout the rice

Mackerel & Orange Salad

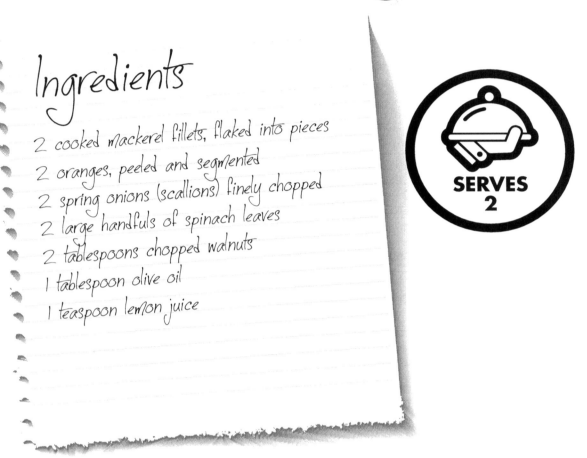

Ingredients

2 cooked mackerel fillets, flaked into pieces

2 oranges, peeled and segmented

2 spring onions (scallions) finely chopped

2 large handfuls of spinach leaves

2 tablespoons chopped walnuts

1 tablespoon olive oil

1 teaspoon lemon juice

SERVES 2

Method

Place the oil and lemon juice in a bowl and mix well. Add the spinach, orange and spring onions (scallions) and coat it in the mixture. Serve the spinach onto plates. Scatter the mackerel over the salad and sprinkle the walnut pieces on top. Serve and eat straight away.

Chicken, Basil & Avocado Salad

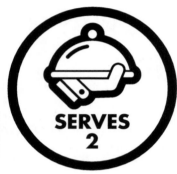

SERVES 2

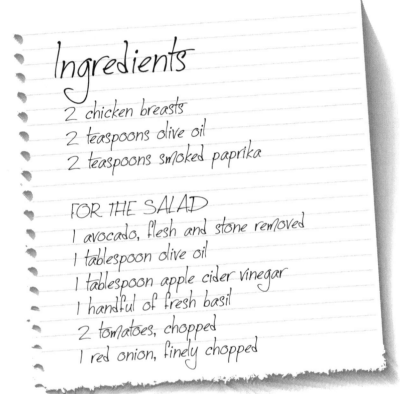

Ingredients

2 chicken breasts
2 teaspoons olive oil
2 teaspoons smoked paprika

FOR THE SALAD
1 avocado, flesh and stone removed
1 tablespoon olive oil
1 tablespoon apple cider vinegar
1 handful of fresh basil
2 tomatoes, chopped
1 red onion, finely chopped

Method

Coat the chicken in the olive oil and sprinkle on the paprika. Place the chicken under a hot grill (broiler) and cook for around 12-14 minutes, until cooked through turning once halfway through. In the meantime, combine the oil, vinegar and basil in a bowl and stir well. Place the tomato, avocado and onion into the dressing and toss the ingredients well. Serve the avocado mixture onto plates and add the chicken breast on top. Eat straight away.

Chicory & Orange Salad

Ingredients

SERVES 2

4 spring onions (scallions, finely chopped)

1 chicory bulb, finely chopped

1 little gem lettuce, chopped

1 fennel bulb, finely chopped

2 tablespoons apple cider vinegar

3 tablespoons olive oil

1 teaspoon mustard

1 large orange, peeled and chopped

Method

Place the lettuce, fennel, chicory, orange and spring onions (scallions) into a bowl. In a separate bowl mix together the olive oil, vinegar and mustard. Pour the dressing over the salad and toss all the ingredients together. Serve and eat straight away.

DINNER

Cajun Salmon With Tomato & Peppers

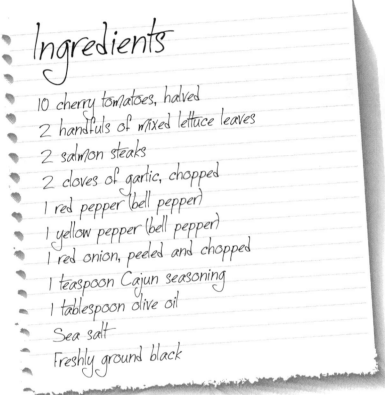

Ingredients

10 cherry tomatoes, halved
2 handfuls of mixed lettuce leaves
2 salmon steaks
2 cloves of garlic, chopped
1 red pepper (bell pepper)
1 yellow pepper (bell pepper)
1 red onion, peeled and chopped
1 teaspoon Cajun seasoning
1 tablespoon olive oil
Sea salt
Freshly ground black

SERVES
2

Method

Coat the salmon in the Cajun seasoning and season with salt and pepper. Heat the oil in a large frying pan and add the salmon. Cook for around 10 minutes, turning once halfway through until completely cooked, pink and opaque throughout. Remove it and set aside, keeping it warm. Add the onion, peppers, garlic and cook for around 5 minutes. Add the tomatoes to the pan and cook for 2 minutes. Scatter the lettuces onto plates and serve the salmon and vegetables on top. Serve and eat straight away.

Baked Cod Ratatouille

Ingredients

4 cod fillets
4 cloves of garlic, chopped
1 yellow pepper (bell pepper)
1 red pepper (bell pepper)
1 large courgette (zucchini)
1 aubergine (eggplant)
1 teaspoon dried mixed herbs
1 tablespoon olive oil
1 large handful of fresh basil leaves, chopped
Sea salt
Freshly ground black pepper

SERVES
4

Method

Place the courgette (zucchini) aubergine (eggplant), peppers, garlic, mixed herbs and oil into an ovenproof roasting dish and toss them well. Season with salt and pepper. Transfer it to the oven and cook at 200C/400F for 25 minutes. Add in half of the fresh basil and stir the vegetables. Place the fish on top of the vegetables. Return it to the oven and cook for 10-12 minutes or until the fish is completely cooked and flakes off.

Szechuan King Prawn Skewers

Ingredients

16 king prawns (shrimps)
8 cherry tomatoes
1 teaspoon Szechuan pepper
1/2 teaspoon sea salt
1 teaspoon olive oil
1/2 teaspoon mild chilli powder
2 cloves of garlic, crushed
1 red onion, cut into wide chunks
1 small bag of salad leaves
1 tablespoon olive oil for drizzling

SERVES 2

Method

Place the salt, garlic, chilli powder and Szechuan pepper into a bowl. Add the prawns (shrimps), tomatoes and onion and coat them in the mixture. Thread the prawns, tomatoes and onion alternately onto skewers. Cook them under a hot grill (broiler), turning during cooking, until the prawns are completely cooked and pink throughout. Serve the salad leaves onto plates and drizzle over a tablespoon of olive oil. Place the skewers on top and enjoy!

Herby Roast Leg of Lamb

Ingredients

2 cloves of garlic, chopped
1 leg of lamb
2 tablespoons fresh rosemary, finely chopped
1 tablespoon olive oil
1/2 teaspoon sea salt
1/2 teaspoon ground black pepper

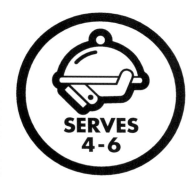

SERVES
4-6

Method

Place the oil, garlic, salt, pepper and rosemary into a blender and blitz until well combined. Make some small cut in the lamb and rub the mixture over the skin and press some into the incisions. Place the lamb in an oven-proof dish or roasting tin and cook until the lamb is done to your liking. It will take around 20 minutes for each 450g (1lb) of meat. Serve with roast potatoes, vegetables or salad.

Rosemary Chicken & Sauerkraut Salad

SERVES 4

Ingredients

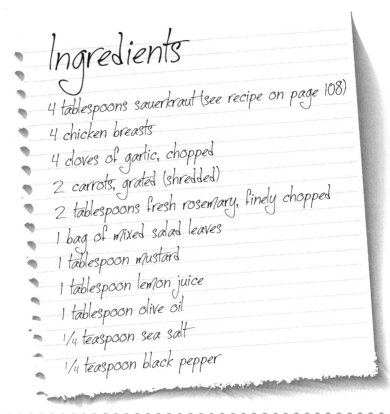

- 4 tablespoons sauerkraut (see recipe on page 108)
- 4 chicken breasts
- 4 cloves of garlic, chopped
- 2 carrots, grated (shredded)
- 2 tablespoons fresh rosemary, finely chopped
- 1 bag of mixed salad leaves
- 1 tablespoon mustard
- 1 tablespoon lemon juice
- 1 tablespoon olive oil
- 1/4 teaspoon sea salt
- 1/4 teaspoon black pepper

Method

Place the oil, garlic, rosemary, lemon juice, mustard salt and pepper into a small bowl and mix well. Transfer half of the dressing to a large bowl and add the chicken breasts. Cover them and allow them to marinade for at least half an hour and longer if you can. Heat a grill (broiler) and place the chicken breasts underneath. Cook for around 5-6 minutes on each side or until the chicken is completely cooked. Scatter the salad leaves and carrots onto plates. Serve the chicken on top and drizzle over the other half of the dressing (make sure not to use any remaining dressing from the uncooked chicken). Add a tablespoon of sauerkraut on the side. Enjoy.

Sweet Potato Fries

Ingredients

4 large sweet potatoes, peeled and cut into strips 1-2cm in thickness

2 tablespoons olive oil

1 teaspoon rosemary (fresh or dried), finely chopped

Sea salt

Freshly ground black pepper

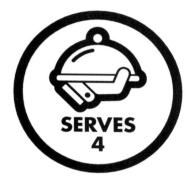

SERVES 4

Method

In a large bowl, coat the sweet potato strips in the olive oil. Sprinkle the rosemary over the potatoes and season with salt and pepper. Line a large backing tray with parchment paper. Scatter the sweet potato over the tray without them overlapping. Use a second tray if you need to. Preheat the oven to 220C/440F and bake the sweet potatoes for 20 minutes or until completely cooked and slightly golden.

Bolognese

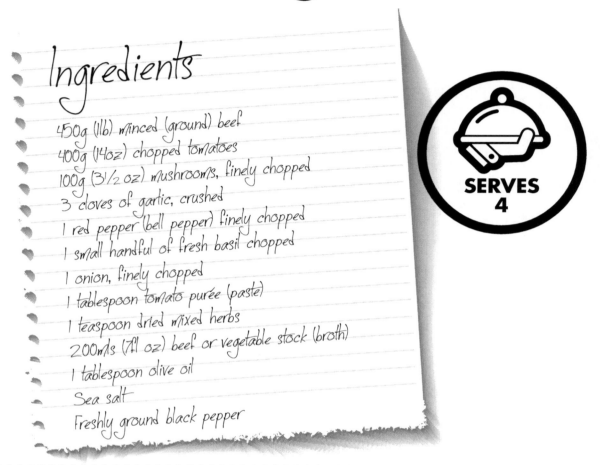

Ingredients

450g (1lb) minced (ground) beef
400g (14oz) chopped tomatoes
100g (3½ oz) mushrooms, finely chopped
3 cloves of garlic, crushed
1 red pepper (bell pepper) finely chopped
1 small handful of fresh basil chopped
1 onion, finely chopped
1 tablespoon tomato purée (paste)
1 teaspoon dried mixed herbs
200mls (7fl oz) beef or vegetable stock (broth)
1 tablespoon olive oil
Sea salt
Freshly ground black pepper

SERVES 4

Method

Heat the olive oil in a large saucepan and beef and cook until the meat browns slightly. Add the onion and garlic and cook until the onion softens. Add the red pepper (bell pepper) and mushrooms. Cook for 2-3 minutes. Pour in the tinned tomatoes, stock (broth), tomato purée and dried herbs. Bring it to the boil, reduce the heat and simmer for 30 minutes. Season with salt and pepper. Simmer for 15-20 minutes. Stir in the basil. Serve with courgette spaghetti or some roast vegetables.

Stuffed Pork Tenderloin

Ingredients

75g (3oz) bacon, chopped
50g (2oz) mushrooms
2 cloves garlic, chopped
1 large pork tenderloin
1 tablespoon ground almonds (almond meal/almond flour)
1 red onion, chopped
1 tablespoon tomato purée (paste)
1 tablespoon fresh basil, chopped
1/2 teaspoon dried oregano
1/2 teaspoon dried basil
1 tablespoon olive oil

SERVES 4

Method

Cut an incision in each piece of pork. Place the almonds, onion, mushrooms, oil, bacon, garlic, basil, tomato purée (paste) and oregano into a food processor and mix until well combined. Spoon the stuffing into the incision in the pork. Heat the olive oil in a pan, and brown the pork fillet. Place it in an ovenproof dish and transfer it to the oven. Cook at 180C/360F for around 1 hour, or until completely cooked through. To check it is completely done, insert a kitchen thermometer which should read 63C/145F. Serve with a heap of roast vegetables.

Butternut Squash & Chicken Casserole

Ingredients

450g (1lb) butternut squash, peeled, deseeded and chopped

75g (3oz) mushrooms, quartered

4 chicken breasts, chopped

1 large leek, chopped

3 cloves of garlic, chopped

2 tablespoons fresh coriander (cilantro), finely chopped

1 teaspoon ground coriander (cilantro)

1 teaspoon ginger

1 litres (1 1/2 pints) chicken stock (broth)

2 teaspoons olive oil

SERVES 4

Method

Heat a teaspoon of oil in a large saucepan, add the chicken and brown it slightly. Remove the chicken and set it aside. Add another teaspoon of oil to the pan and add the squash and cook for around 6 minutes until it has softened. Add the leek, garlic, ground coriander (cilantro) and ginger and cook for 2 minutes. Add in the stock (broth), mushrooms and chicken and cook for 10 minutes, making sure the chicken is cooked through. Stir in the fresh coriander (cilantro) and serve.

Roast Vegetables

Ingredients

150g (5oz) cherry tomatoes, halved

150g (5oz) button mushrooms

1 large onion, chopped

1 courgette (zucchini), chopped

3 celery stalks, chopped

3 cloves of garlic, peeled and chopped

2 carrots, peeled and roughly

1 whole beetroot, washed and roughly chopped

1 butternut squash, peeled and cut into chunks

1 teaspoon dried thyme

1 teaspoon dried oregano

1 large handful of fresh parsley

1 tablespoon olive oil

Sea salt

Freshly ground black pepper

SERVES 4

Method

Place all of the vegetables into an ovenproof dish. Sprinkle in the dried herbs, garlic and olive oil and toss all of the ingredients together. Season with salt and pepper. Transfer them to an oven, preheated to 180C/360F and cook for 30-40 minutes or until all of the vegetables are softened and cooked through. Scatter in the fresh parsley just before serving.

Mildly Spiced Salmon Kebabs

SERVES 4

Ingredients

- 4 salmon fillets, cut into thick chunks
- 3 spring onions (scallions), finely chopped
- 1 courgette (zucchini), thickly sliced
- 1 teaspoon cayenne pepper
- 1 teaspoon ground cumin
- 1 teaspoon ground coriander (cilantro)
- 2 cardamom pods, seeds only
- 1 tablespoon lemon juice
- 2 teaspoons olive oil
- Salt and freshly ground pepper

Method

In a bowl, combine the cayenne, cumin, coriander (cilantro), spring onions (scallions), cardamom and lemon juice. In a separate bowl, add the olive oil, salt and pepper and coat the salmon in the mixture. Thread the salmon chunks and courgette (zucchini) onto skewers. Place them under a hot grill (broiler) and cook for around 3 minutes on each side or until the fish is opaque and completely cooked through. Serve with the dressing and a heap of green leafy salad.

Potato & Egg Salad

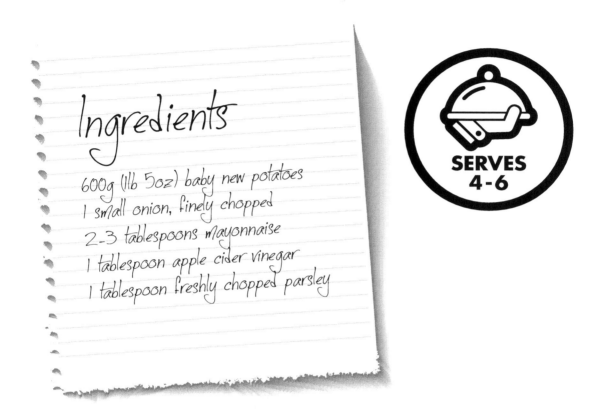

Ingredients

600g (1lb 5oz) baby new potatoes
1 small onion, finely chopped
2-3 tablespoons mayonnaise
1 tablespoon apple cider vinegar
1 tablespoon freshly chopped parsley

SERVES 4-6

Method

Cook the potatoes in salted water for 15-20 minutes or until they are cooked through. Drain them and allow them to cool. Roughly chop the potatoes and add them to a large bowl along with the onion. In a small bowl combine the mayonnaise, vinegar and parsley. Stir the mayo into the potatoes. Chill before serving.

Chilli Salmon & Celeriac Coleslaw

SERVES 2

Ingredients

200g (7oz) celeriac, peeled and grated (shredded)

2 carrot, grated (shredded)

2 salmon fillets

1 onion, grated (shredded)

½ teaspoon chilli powder

1 tablespoon mayonnaise

2 teaspoons apple cider vinegar

2 teaspoons wholegrain mustard

2 teaspoons olive oil

Method

Place the olive oil and chilli into a bowl and stir well. Coat the salmon fillets in the chilli oil mixture. Place the salmon under a hot grill (broiler) and cook for around 15 minutes or until completely cooked, turning them halfway through cooking. In the meantime, place the mayonnaise, vinegar and mustard into a bowl and mix well. Add the celeriac, carrot and onion to the mayonnaise and coat the vegetables well. Serve onto plates along with the salmon. Eat straight away.

CONDIMENTS & DIPS

Garlic Mayonnaise

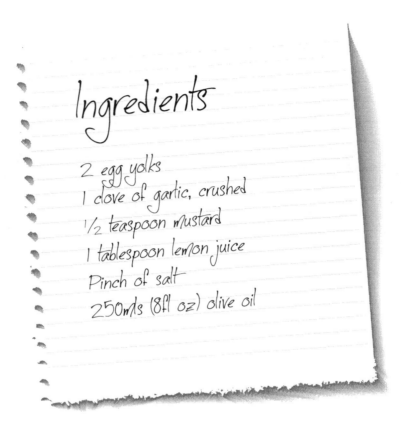

Ingredients

2 egg yolks
1 clove of garlic, crushed
½ teaspoon mustard
1 tablespoon lemon juice
Pinch of salt
250mls (8fl oz) olive oil

Method

Place the eggs, garlic, mustard, salt and lemon juice into a food processor and combine them. If your blender has a funnel, slowly pour in the oil until it emulsifies. If it doesn't have a funnel, slowly add the oil while processing at a very slow speed. Store the mayonnaise in a lidded jar in the fridge

Basic Vinaigrette

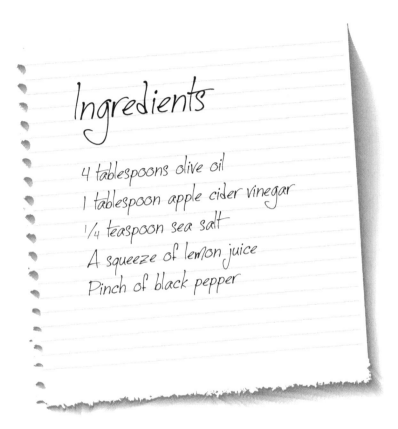

Ingredients

4 tablespoons olive oil
1 tablespoon apple cider vinegar
1/4 teaspoon sea salt
A squeeze of lemon juice
Pinch of black pepper

Method

Mix the ingredients together in a jar or bow land keep chilled until ready to use.

Tomato Vinaigrette

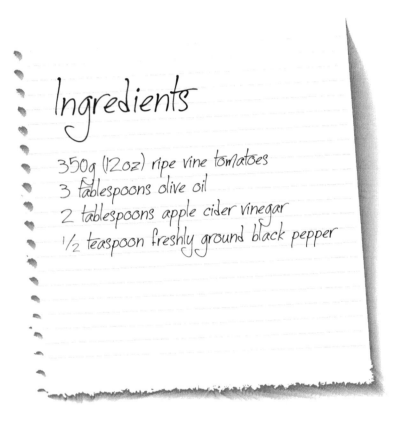

Ingredients

- 350g (12oz) ripe vine tomatoes
- 3 tablespoons olive oil
- 2 tablespoons apple cider vinegar
- 1/2 teaspoon freshly ground black pepper

Method

Prepare a bowl of hot water and a bowl of iced water. Gently, place the tomatoes into the hot water and leave them for around a minute when the skin should pucker. Carefully remove them and place them in the iced water. The skin should now peel off easily. Place the tomatoes, oil, vinegar and black pepper into a blender and blitz until smooth. Serve as a salad dressing or with meat, chicken and fish dishes.

Coriander Salsa

Ingredients

4 ripe tomatoes, deseeded and chopped
1 red pepper (bell pepper), finely chopped
1 small red onion, finely chopped
A large handful of fresh coriander (cilantro) leaves, chopped
Squeeze of lemon juice
Sea salt
Freshly ground black pepper

Method

Place the red pepper (bell pepper) under a hot grill (broiler) and cook until the skin blisters. Place the pepper in a bowl and cover with plastic wrap for 2 minutes to loosen the skin then peel it. Discard the skin and chop the flesh. Combine the pepper in a bowl with the onion, tomatoes, coriander (cilantro) and lemon juice. Season with salt and pepper. Serve with meat, chicken and fish dishes or even alongside salads.

Basil & Garlic Pesto

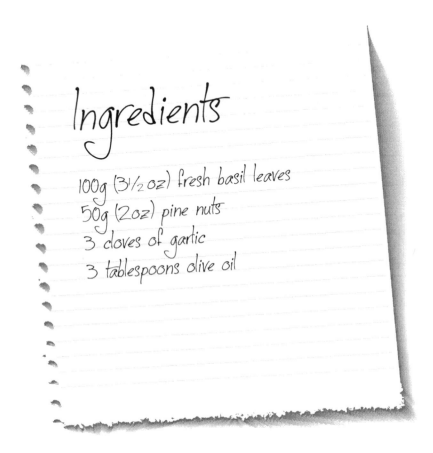

Ingredients

100g (3½ oz) fresh basil leaves
50g (2oz) pine nuts
3 cloves of garlic
3 tablespoons olive oil

Method

Place all of the ingredients into a blender and process until smooth. If the pesto is thicker than you would like, add a little extra oil. Store in the fridge until ready to use as a marinade or dressing or even as a dip.

Guacamole

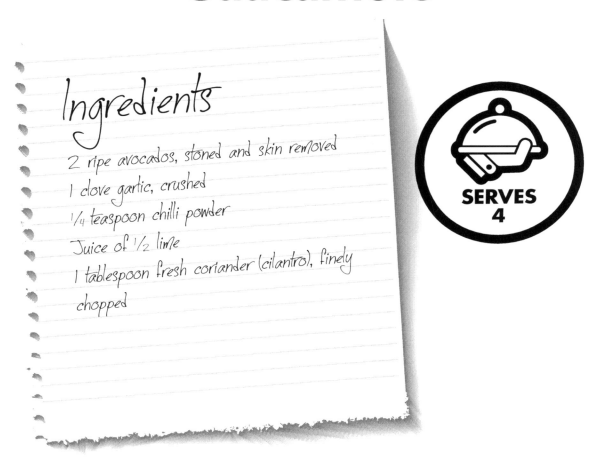

Ingredients

2 ripe avocados, stoned and skin removed

1 clove garlic, crushed

1/4 teaspoon chilli powder

Juice of 1/2 lime

1 tablespoon fresh coriander (cilantro), finely
chopped

**SERVES
4**

Method

Place all the ingredients into a bowl or a food processor if you'd prefer and combine the
ingredients until smooth. Serve as a dip or an addition to salads, chilli and chicken dishes.

Bone Broth

Ingredients

1 chicken carcass (leftover from roast chicken is ideal)
1 leek, roughly chopped
1 onion, roughly chopped
1 carrot, roughly chopped
2 bay leaves
1/2 teaspoon black pepper
1/2 teaspoon sea salt
3 litres (4.5 pints) water

Method

Place all of the ingredients into a large saucepan. Bring it to the boil, reduce the heat and allow it to simmer gently for 1 hour. Using a sieve or colander, strain off the liquid into a large jug or bowl. Discard the bones and vegetables. Use the broth as a base stock for soups, casseroles or curries.

Stage 2 Recipes

BREAKFAST

Spiced Peach Smoothie

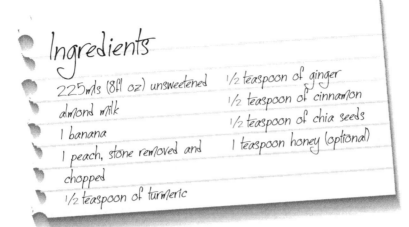

Ingredients

225mls (8fl oz) unsweetened almond milk

1 banana

1 peach, stone removed and chopped

1/2 teaspoon of turmeric

1/2 teaspoon of ginger

1/2 teaspoon of cinnamon

1/2 teaspoon of chia seeds

1 teaspoon honey (optional)

SERVES 1

Method

Place all of the ingredients into a blender and process until smooth and creamy. Enjoy!

Ginger & Avocado Cream Smoothie

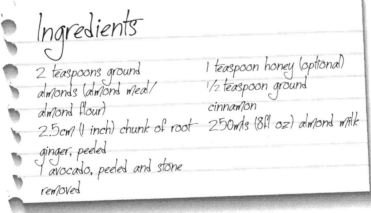

Ingredients

2 teaspoons ground almonds (almond meal/ almond flour)

2.5cm (1 inch) chunk of root ginger, peeled

1 avocado, peeled and stone removed

1 teaspoon honey (optional)

1/2 teaspoon ground cinnamon

250mls (8fl oz) almond milk

SERVES 1

Method

Place all of the ingredients into a food processor and blitz until smooth and creamy. Serve straight away.

Nutty Yogurt Smoothie

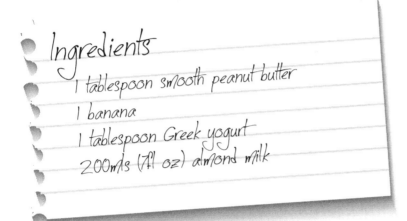

Ingredients
- 1 tablespoon smooth peanut butter
- 1 banana
- 1 tablespoon Greek yogurt
- 200mls (7fl oz) almond milk

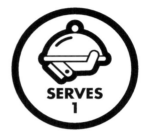

SERVES
1

Method

Place all the ingredients into a blender and process until smooth and creamy.
Add a few ice cubes. Enjoy straight away.

Pistachio, Pear and Passion Fruit Yogurt

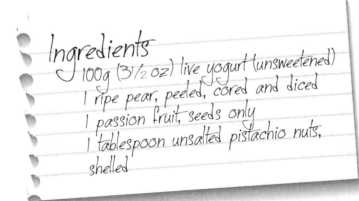

Ingredients
- 100g (3½ oz) live yogurt (unsweetened)
- 1 ripe pear, peeled, cored and diced
- 1 passion fruit, seeds only
- 1 tablespoon unsalted pistachio nuts, shelled

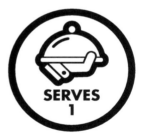

SERVES
1

Method

Spoon the yogurt into a serving bowl and stir in the pear and pistachio nuts.
Sprinkle the passion fruit over the top. Eat straight away.

Coconut Granola

Ingredients

- 125g (4oz) almonds, chopped
- 125g (4oz) chopped walnuts
- 125g (4oz) chopped pecans
- 50g (2oz) unsweetened coconut flakes
- 50g (2oz) pumpkin seeds
- 50g (2oz) sesame seeds
- 50g (2oz) ground flaxseeds (linseeds)
- 120mls (4fl oz) coconut oil, melted
- 2 tablespoons honey
- 1 teaspoon cinnamon
- 1/2 teaspoon sea salt

SERVES
?

Method

Line a baking tray with parchment paper. In a bowl mix together the honey, coconut oil, cinnamon and salt. Place the nuts and seeds into a large bowl and coat them in the oil mixture. Scatter the ingredients evenly onto the baking tray. Transfer it to the oven, preheated to 150C/200F and cook for 15 minutes then stir the granola. Cook for another 15 minutes or until golden. Allow it to cool then store it in an airtight container. You can eat it on its own as a snack or with nut milk or live yogurt.

Turmeric & Coriander Eggs

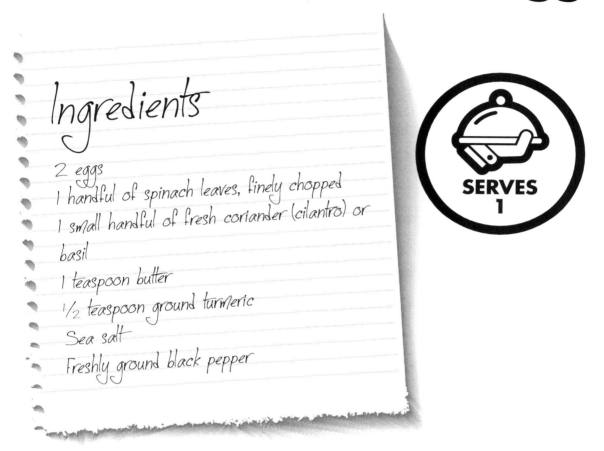

Ingredients

2 eggs

1 handful of spinach leaves, finely chopped

1 small handful of fresh coriander (cilantro) or basil

1 teaspoon butter

1/2 teaspoon ground turmeric

Sea salt

Freshly ground black pepper

SERVES 1

Method

Break the eggs into a bowl, sprinkle in the turmeric and season with salt and pepper. Heat the butter in a frying pan, add in the spinach and cook for around 1 minute or until wilted. Pour the egg mixture into the pan and sprinkle in half of the coriander (cilantro). Stir constantly, scrambling the eggs until they are set. Sprinkle on the remaining herbs and serve.

Paprika & Herb Mug Muffin

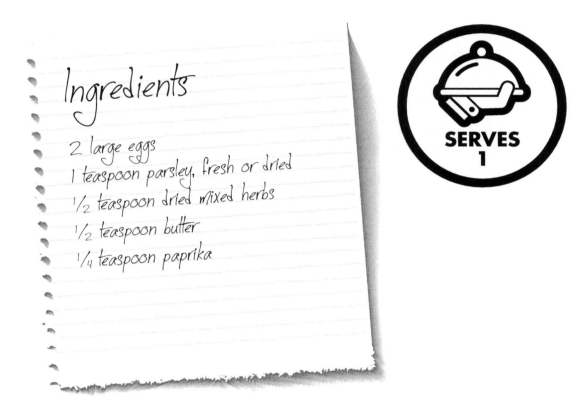

SERVES 1

Ingredients

2 large eggs
1 teaspoon parsley, fresh or dried
1/2 teaspoon dried mixed herbs
1/2 teaspoon butter
1/4 teaspoon paprika

Method

Crack the eggs into a large mug and beat them. Add in the butter, herbs and paprika. Place the mug in a microwave and cook on full power for 30 seconds. Stir the egg mixture. Return it to the microwave for another 30 seconds, stir again then cook for another 30-60 seconds or until the egg is completely cooked. Eat it straight from the mug for a fast and tasty breakfast. You can try adding other ingredients like tomatoes, spring onions (scallions) and basil.

LUNCH

Stilton & Asparagus

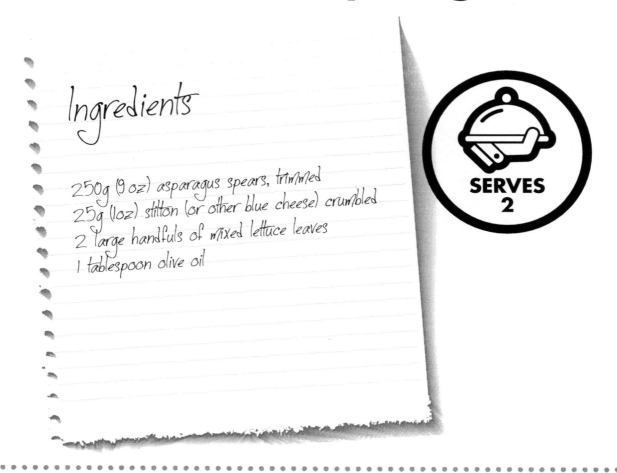

Ingredients

250g (9 oz) asparagus spears, trimmed
25g (1oz) stilton (or other blue cheese) crumbled
2 large handfuls of mixed lettuce leaves
1 tablespoon olive oil

SERVES 2

Method

Heat the olive oil in a griddle pan or a large frying pan. Add the asparagus to the pan and cook for around 4 minutes, turning to ensure even cooking. Scatter the lettuce leaves onto plates and serve the asparagus on top. Sprinkle the cheese onto the asparagus. Eat straight away.

Parsnip Soup

Ingredients

- 75g (3oz) stilton cheese, or other blue cheese
- 4 large parsnips, peeled and chopped
- 2 cloves of garlic
- 1 large onion, peeled and chopped
- 1 tablespoon apple cider vinegar
- 1 tablespoon olive oil
- 900mls (1 ½ pints) chicken or vegetable stock (broth)

SERVES 4

Method

Heat the oil in a saucepan, add the onion and cook for 5 minutes. Add in the chopped parsnips, stock (broth) and garlic and cook for 15-20 minutes or until the parsnip has softened. Stir in the vinegar and half of the blue cheese. Using a hand blender or food processor blitz the soup until smooth. Serve with some of the remaining cheese scattered on top.

High Protein Bread

Ingredients

200g (7oz) ground almonds (almond meal/almond flour)

100g (3½oz) ground linseeds (flaxseeds)

5 eggs

3 tablespoon coconut flour

2 tablespoons raw honey

1 tablespoon apple cider vinegar

1 tablespoon coconut oil

½ teaspoon baking soda

⅓ teaspoon sea salt

Method

Grease and line a 8x4 inch loaf tin. Place the ground almonds (almond meal/almond flour), coconut flour, ground linseeds (flaxseeds), salt and baking soda into a bowl and mix well. Add in the eggs, oil, honey and vinegar and mix until thoroughly combined. Scoop the mixture into the loaf tin. Bake in an oven, preheated to 350F for 30 minutes. Test the centre using a skewer to check if it is cooked in middle and give it another few minutes if it needs it. Allow it to cool then store in an airtight container.

Chicken & Roquefort Soup

Ingredients

350g (12oz) leftover chicken, chopped
50g (2oz) Roquefort cheese (or other blue cheese)
4 stalks of celery, chopped
1 small courgette (zucchini), chopped
1 tablespoon olive oil
1 onion, chopped
1 leek, chopped
1 tablespoon fresh parsley
900mls (1 ½ pints) chicken stock (broth)

SERVES
4

Method

Heat the oil in a large saucepan, add the leek, celery, courgette (zucchini) and onion and cook for 5 minutes. Add the chicken stock (broth), bring it to the boil, reduce the heat and cook for 10 minutes, stirring occasionally. Using a hand blender or food processor blitz the soup until smooth. Add in the chicken and warm it through. Stir in the parsley and serve into bowls with a scattering of blue cheese on top.

Smoked Salmon, Pears & Walnut Salad

SERVES 4

Ingredients

50g (2oz) blue cheese, crumbled (optional)

350g (12 oz) smoked salmon

50g (2oz) walnuts, roughly chopped

2 pears, peeled, cored and diced

1 bag of fresh watercress

2 tablespoons olive oil

1 tablespoon apple cider vinegar

Sea salt

Freshly ground black pepper

Method

In a small bowl, combine the oil, vinegar salt and pepper. Toss the watercress in the dressing and serve it onto plates. Lay the smoked salmon onto the watercress and scatter the pear, walnuts and blue cheese (if using) over the top.

Cauliflower Mash

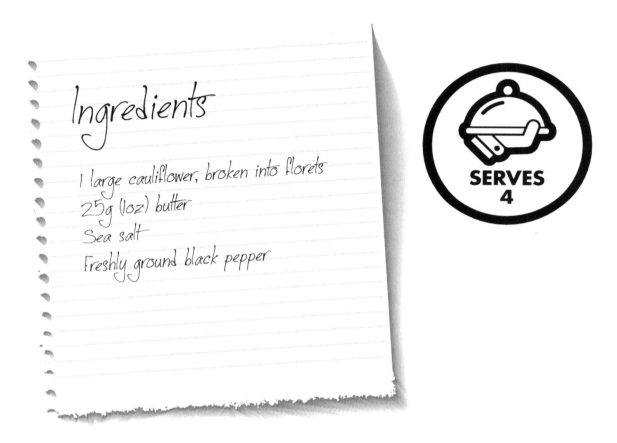

Ingredients

1 large cauliflower, broken into florets
25g (1oz) butter
Sea salt
Freshly ground black pepper

SERVES 4

Method

Place the cauliflower into a steamer and cook for 8-10 minutes or until tender. Use a hand blender or food processor and blitz until smooth. If you're using a food processor, let it cool slightly first. Add the butter (if using), salt and pepper and combine until it becomes smooth. Use cauliflower mash as an alternative to pasta, rice and starchy carbs.

Egg Fried 'Rice'

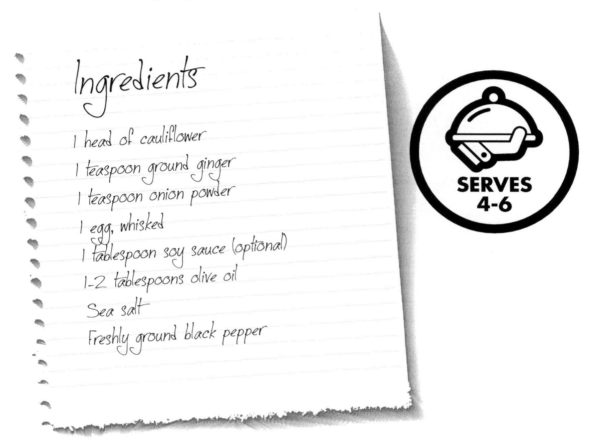

SERVES 4-6

Ingredients

1 head of cauliflower

1 teaspoon ground ginger

1 teaspoon onion powder

1 egg, whisked

1 tablespoon soy sauce (optional)

1-2 tablespoons olive oil

Sea salt

Freshly ground black pepper

Method

Place the cauliflower into a food processor and chop until fine grains. Heat the oil in a frying pan. Stir in the ginger, onion powder and the cauliflower grains are soft. Cook for around 6 minutes or until softened. Towards the end of cooking, move the cauliflower to one side of the pan, making a space for the egg. Pour the egg into the space and stir it briskly with a fork breaking it up. Once it's cooked stir it throughout the rice along with the soy sauce (optional). Season with salt and pepper and serve.

Thai Chicken Burgers

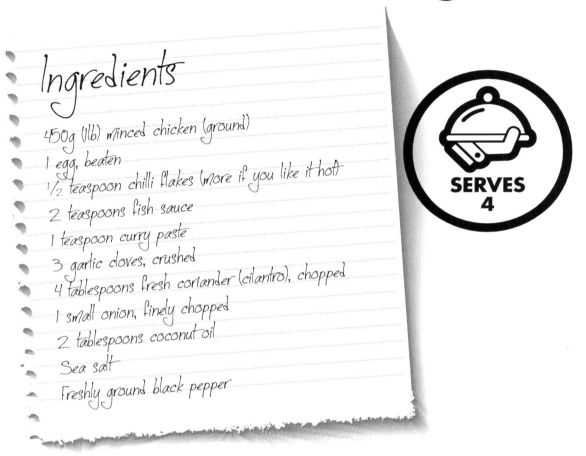

Ingredients

450g (1lb) minced chicken (ground)

1 egg, beaten

1/2 teaspoon chilli flakes (more if you like it hot)

2 teaspoons fish sauce

1 teaspoon curry paste

3 garlic cloves, crushed

4 tablespoons fresh coriander (cilantro), chopped

1 small onion, finely chopped

2 tablespoons coconut oil

Sea salt

Freshly ground black pepper

SERVES 4

Method

In a large bowl, combine the chicken with the garlic, onion, chilli, curry paste, fish sauce and coriander (cilantro). Add in the egg to bind all the ingredients together. Season with salt and pepper. Mix the ingredients together well. Divide the mixture into 4 and form into burger shapes. Heat the coconut oil in a frying pan. Place the burgers in the pan and cook for around 7- 8 minutes on either side until the burgers are cooked through. Serve them in iceberg or romaine lettuce leaves instead of a bread bun. Add a dollop of mayonnaise or guacamole.

Chicken & Toasted Pine Nut Salad

Ingredients

- 8 pitted olives, halved
- 4 cooked chicken breasts, sliced
- 4 tablespoons pine nuts, roughly chopped
- 2 avocados, peeled, stone removed and thickly sliced
- 2 little gem lettuce, chopped
- 2 tomatoes, chopped
- 1 bag of mixed lettuce leaves
- 1 small handful of fresh basil leaves, chopped
- 1 tablespoon balsamic vinegar
- 2 tablespoons olive oil
- 1 tablespoon apple cider vinegar
- Sea salt
- Freshly ground black pepper

SERVES 4

Method

Place the pine nuts in a frying pan and dry fry them until they are slightly golden. In a bowl, combine the vinegars, oil and season with salt and pepper. Add the lettuce, olives, tomatoes and avocado to the dressing and toss the ingredients well. Serve the salad onto plates. Lay the sliced chicken on top. Scatter the pine nuts and basil over the salads.

Egg Mayo Chicory Shells

Ingredients

4 large eggs, hard-boiled, cooled and peeled

1 teaspoon Dijon mustard

2 tablespoons mayonnaise

1 tablespoon plain (unflavoured) live Greek yogurt

1 teaspoon fresh parsley, chopped

1 teaspoon fresh chives, chopped

1 chicory, separated into leaves

1/2 teaspoon sea salt

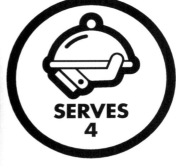

SERVES 4

Method

Place the eggs, mayonnaise, yogurt, mustard and salt into a bowl and mash the eggs in with the other ingredients. Stir in the chives. Spoon the mixture into the chicory leaves. Sprinkle with parsley and place them on a serving plate.

Radish Tzatziki

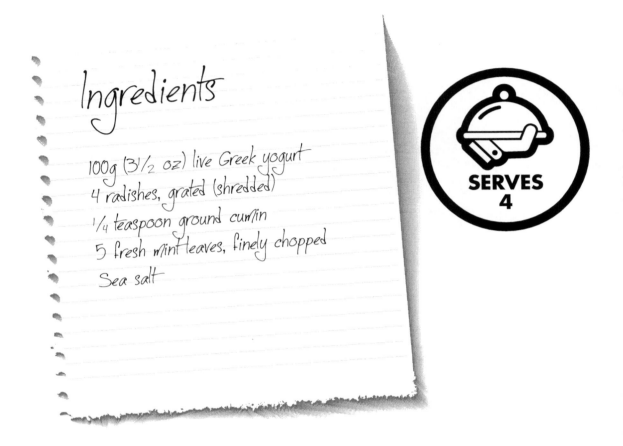

Ingredients

100g (3½ oz) live Greek yogurt
4 radishes, grated (shredded)
¼ teaspoon ground cumin
5 fresh mint leaves, finely chopped
Sea salt

SERVES 4

Method

Place all of the ingredients into a bowl and mix well. Serve as an accompaniment to meat, chicken, fish and curry dishes or use it as a dip with chopped vegetables.

DINNER

Prawn & Lobster Cocktail

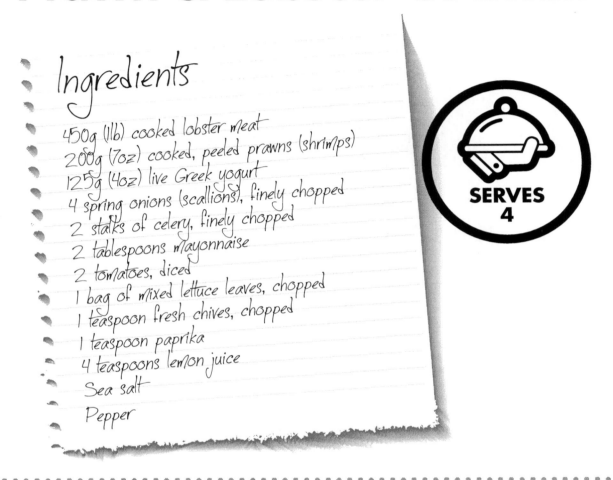

Ingredients

450g (1lb) cooked lobster meat
200g (7oz) cooked, peeled prawns (shrimps)
125g (4oz) live Greek yogurt
4 spring onions (scallions), finely chopped
2 stalks of celery, finely chopped
2 tablespoons mayonnaise
2 tomatoes, diced
1 bag of mixed lettuce leaves, chopped
1 teaspoon fresh chives, chopped
1 teaspoon paprika
4 teaspoons lemon juice
Sea salt
Pepper

SERVES 4

Method

Place the mayonnaise, yogurt, celery, spring onions (scallions), lemon juice, chives and paprika into a bowl and mix well. Stir in the prawns (shrimps) and lobster and coat them in the dressing. Season with salt and pepper. Place the lettuce and tomatoes into serving bowls or plates and spoon the seafood mixture on top. Chill before serving.

Steak Salad With Lemon & Chive Dressing

SERVES 2

Ingredients

75g (3oz) live Greek yogurt
2 beef steaks
2 large handfuls of mixed lettuce leaves
1 red pepper (bell pepper), finely chopped
1 small bunch of chives, finely chopped
2 teaspoons lemon juice
3 teaspoons mayonnaise
1 teaspoon olive oil
Sea salt
Freshly ground black pepper

Method

Sprinkle a little salt and pepper onto the steak. Heat the oil in a frying pan and cooked until it's done to your liking. Allow the steak to rest. In the meantime, place the yogurt, chives, lemon juice and mayonnaise in a bowl and combine the ingredients. Season with salt and pepper.

Thinly slice the steak. Scatter the lettuce and red pepper (bell pepper) onto plates. Serve the steak on top and spoon the dressing over the salad. Enjoy straight away.

Smokey Bean & Mushroom Stew

Ingredients

- 400g (14oz) black-eyed peas
- 400g (14oz) haricot beans
- 400g (14oz) tinned tomatoes, chopped
- 225g (8oz) button mushrooms, halved
- 2 carrots, peeled and diced
- 3 garlic cloves, chopped
- 2 onions, chopped
- 1 red pepper (bell pepper), deseeded and chopped
- 1 tablespoon smoked paprika
- 1 tablespoon tomato purée (paste)
- 1 red chilli, finely chopped
- 1 large handful of parsley
- 600mls (1 pint) stock (broth)
- 2 tablespoons tamari or soy sauce
- 1 tablespoon olive oil

SERVES 4

Method

Heat the oil in a saucepan, add the mushrooms, carrots, onions and garlic and cook for 5-6 minutes until they have softened. Stir in the chilli, haricot beans, black-eyed peas, tomatoes, red pepper (bell pepper), purée (paste), paprika and tamari/soy sauce and cook for 5 minutes. Pour in the stock (broth) and simmer for around 20 minutes. Stir in the fresh parsley. Serve on its own or with cauliflower rice and a dollop of guacamole.

Chicken Tikka & Roast Vegetables

Ingredients

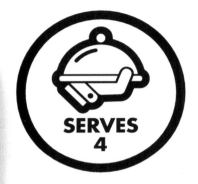

SERVES 4

FOR THE VEGETABLES:

1 large aubergine (eggplant) cut into thick chunks

4 large tomatoes, de-seeded and cut into chunks

1 red pepper (bell pepper)

1 yellow pepper (bell pepper)

1 tablespoon olive oil

1 handful fresh coriander (cilantro), chopped

FOR THE CHICKEN:

4 chicken breasts

2.5cm (1 inch) chunk of fresh ginger root, finely chopped

1 clove of garlic, crushed

1 teaspoon chilli powder

1/2 teaspoon sea salt

1/2 teaspoon turmeric

125g (4oz) plain (unflavoured) Greek yogurt

1 tablespoon olive oil

Juice of 1 lemon

Method

For the chicken; place the chilli, salt, oil, turmeric, ginger, garlic, yogurt and lemon juice in a bowl and stir it well. Coat the chicken in the mixture. Place the vegetables in a large ovenproof dish and coat them in a tablespoon of olive oil. Make a space in the centre of the dish for the chicken breasts or place them on top. Transfer the dish to the oven and cook at 180C/360F for around 35 to 40 minutes or until the chicken is cooked through. Scatter the chopped coriander (cilantro) over the top and serve.

Pomegranate & Red Pepper Chicken

SERVES 4

Ingredients

100g (3½ oz) passata or chopped tomatoes

4 handfuls of fresh spinach leaves

4 chicken breasts

2 red peppers (bell peppers), chopped

Seeds from 2 pomegranates

2 onions, chopped

2 tablespoons balsamic vinegar

2 tablespoons olive oil

½ teaspoon ground cinnamon

1 handful of fresh coriander (cilantro) chopped

Method

Place the olive oil, vinegar, passata/tomatoes and cinnamon into a bowl and mix well.
Coat the chicken thoroughly in the mixture. Scatter the onions and peppers into an
ovenproof dish and lay the chicken mixture on top. Cook in the oven for around 35
minutes at 200C/400F. Sprinkle on the coriander (cilantro) and pomegranate seeds.
Scatter the spinach onto each of the plates and serve the chicken and vegetables on top.

Beef Stroganoff

Ingredients

450g (1lb) beef sirloin, sliced
300g (11oz) plain yogurt
250g (9 oz) mushrooms, sliced
2 tablespoons paprika
2 tablespoons olive oil
1 onion, finely chopped
Salt & pepper
A handful of fresh parsley, finely chopped for garnish

SERVES 4

Method

Heat a tablespoon of oil in a pan, add the mushrooms and onions and cook for around 5 minutes until they soften. Remove them from the pan and keep them warm. Coat the beef in the paprika. Heat a tablespoon of oil and add the beef. Cook it for a few minutes, stirring occasionally until the beef is brown. Return the onions and mushrooms to the pan. Add in the yogurt and warm the casserole through. Season with salt and pepper and sprinkle in the parsley. Serve with cauliflower rice.

Haddock & Minty Pea Purée

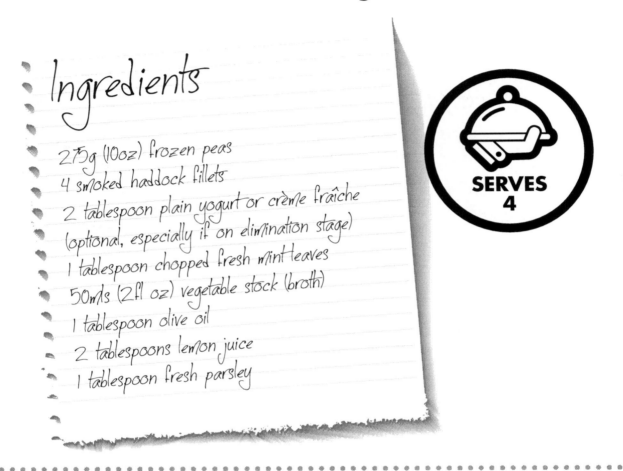

Ingredients

- 275g (10oz) frozen peas
- 4 smoked haddock fillets
- 2 tablespoon plain yogurt or crème fraîche (optional, especially if on elimination stage)
- 1 tablespoon chopped fresh mint leaves
- 50mls (2fl oz) vegetable stock (broth)
- 1 tablespoon olive oil
- 2 tablespoons lemon juice
- 1 tablespoon fresh parsley

SERVES 4

Method

Place the oil, lemon juice and parsley into a small bowl and stir well. Place the haddock in an ovenproof dish and drizzle the oil mixture over the top making sure it's well coated. Preheat the oven to 180C/360F and bake the fish for around 20 minutes or until it is flaky and tender. In the meantime, place the peas in a saucepan with hot water and bring them to the boil. Add the stock (broth) to the peas and the mint and yogurt/crème fraîche (if using). Use a hand blender and purée the pea mixture until smooth. Spoon the peas onto plates and serve the fish on top. Enjoy.

Honey & Lemon Chicken Drumsticks

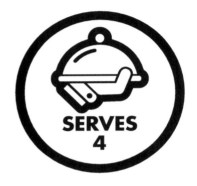

SERVES 4

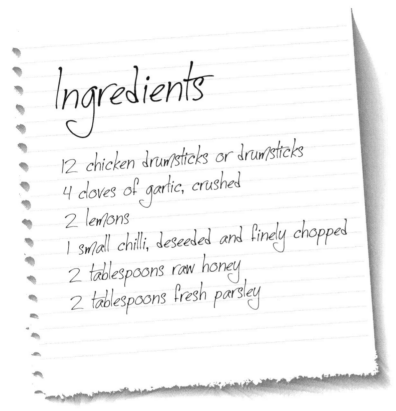

Ingredients

12 chicken drumsticks or drumsticks
4 cloves of garlic, crushed
2 lemons
1 small chilli, deseeded and finely chopped
2 tablespoons raw honey
2 tablespoons fresh parsley

Method

Cut the lemons in half and squeeze the juice into a large bowl. Slice the lemon skins and scatter them in an ovenproof dish. Add the garlic, chilli and honey to the lemon juice. Coat the chicken drumsticks lemon mixture and let them marinade for at least an hour. Lay the chicken on top of the lemon skins. Transfer it to the oven and cook at 200C/400F for 40-45 minutes or until the chicken is completely cooked through. Sprinkle with parsley and serve with salads or cauliflower rice.

Cobb Salad

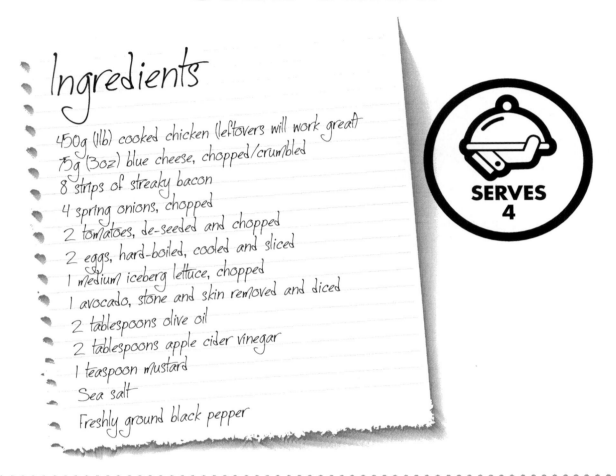

Ingredients

450g (1lb) cooked chicken (leftovers will work great)

75g (3oz) blue cheese, chopped/crumbled

8 strips of streaky bacon

4 spring onions, chopped

2 tomatoes, de-seeded and chopped

2 eggs, hard-boiled, cooled and sliced

1 medium iceberg lettuce, chopped

1 avocado, stone and skin removed and diced

2 tablespoons olive oil

2 tablespoons apple cider vinegar

1 teaspoon mustard

Sea salt

Freshly ground black pepper

SERVES 4

Method

Place the bacon under a hot grill (broiler) and cook on each side until crisp and golden. Chop it and set it aside. Scatter the chopped lettuce onto plates. Serve the chicken, avocado, eggs, bacon, spring onions (scallions) and blue cheese decoratively in lines on top of the lettuce. Combine the oil, vinegar, mustard, salt and pepper in a bowl and mix well. Drizzle the dressing over the top. Eat straight away.

DESSERTS & SWEET TREATS

Chocolate Bean Brownies

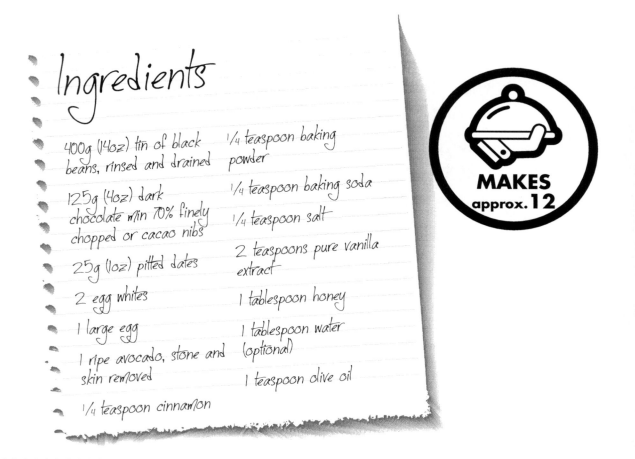

Ingredients

400g (14oz) tin of black beans, rinsed and drained

125g (4oz) dark chocolate min 70% finely chopped or cacao nibs

25g (1oz) pitted dates

2 egg whites

1 large egg

1 ripe avocado, stone and skin removed

1/4 teaspoon cinnamon

1/4 teaspoon baking powder

1/4 teaspoon baking soda

1/4 teaspoon salt

2 teaspoons pure vanilla extract

1 tablespoon honey

1 tablespoon water (optional)

1 teaspoon olive oil

MAKES approx. 12

Method

Place all of the ingredients, except the chocolate into a blender and blitz until smooth. If the mixture seems very thick, add the tablespoon of water if you need to. Just add a teaspoon or two or water. Add the chocolate to the ingredients and mix well. Grease and line a baking tin and pour in the mixture. Transfer it to an oven preheated to 180C/360F for around 25 minutes. Once it has cooled cut it into bars. Store in an airtight container in the fridge or eat straight away.

Lemon Coconut Fingers

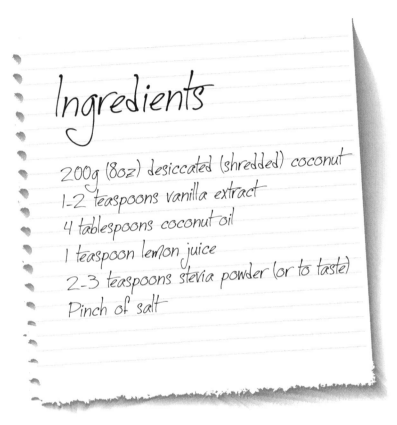

Ingredients

200g (8oz) desiccated (shredded) coconut
1-2 teaspoons vanilla extract
4 tablespoons coconut oil
1 teaspoon lemon juice
2-3 teaspoons stevia powder (or to taste)
Pinch of salt

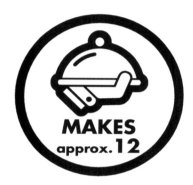

MAKES
approx. 12

Method

Place all of the ingredients into a food processor and blitz until smooth. Line a small baking tin with greaseproof paper then spoon the coconut into the tin, pressing it into the sides and smoothing it out. Chill in the fridge for 2 hours. Slice the coconut mixture into fingers and store them in an airtight container in the fridge until ready to use.

Cherry Chocolate & Chia Dessert

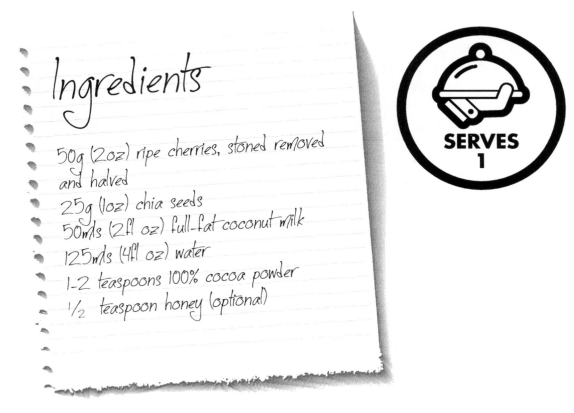

Ingredients

50g (2oz) ripe cherries, stoned removed and halved
25g (1oz) chia seeds
50mls (2fl oz) full-fat coconut milk
125mls (4fl oz) water
1-2 teaspoons 100% cocoa powder
½ teaspoon honey (optional)

SERVES 1

Method

Place the chia seeds, honey, and cocoa powder into a bowl and stir in the water and coconut milk. Transfer the mixture to a serving bowl. Cover it and place it in the fridge for 20-30 minutes. Serve with the cherries scattered over the top.

Coconut Chai Latte

Ingredients

400mls (14fl oz) coconut milk
400mls (14fl oz) water
1 star anise
1 teaspoon turmeric
1 teaspoon ground nutmeg
1 teaspoon ground ginger
1 teaspoon ground cinnamon
1/2 teaspoon ground cloves
4 cardamom pods
3 teaspoons honey (or to taste) optional
Pinch of salt

**SERVES
4**

Method

Place the water, honey, salt, cinnamon, ginger, star anise, turmeric, nutmeg, cloves
and cardamom in a saucepan, bring it to the boil. Reduce the heat and simmer for
5 minutes. Strain the liquid through a sieve to remove and return it to the saucepan.
Add the coconut milk to the saucepan and warm it through. Pour into a heatproof
glass or a cup. Drink it straight away.

Mango Lassi

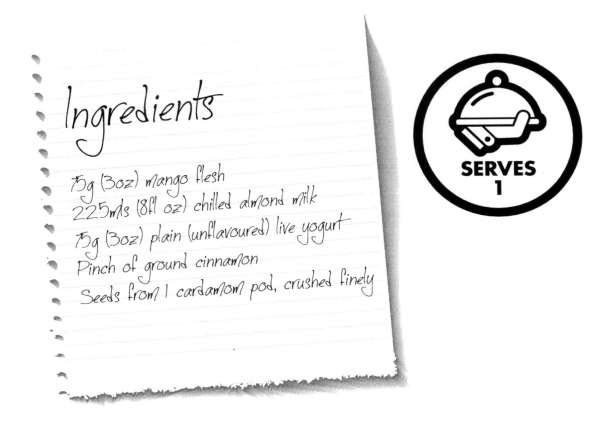

Ingredients

75g (3oz) mango flesh
225mls (8fl oz) chilled almond milk
75g (3oz) plain (unflavoured) live yogurt
Pinch of ground cinnamon
Seeds from 1 cardamom pod, crushed finely

**SERVES
1**

Method

Place all of the ingredients into a blender and blitz until smooth and creamy. Enjoy it straight away.

Strawberry Yogurt Lollies

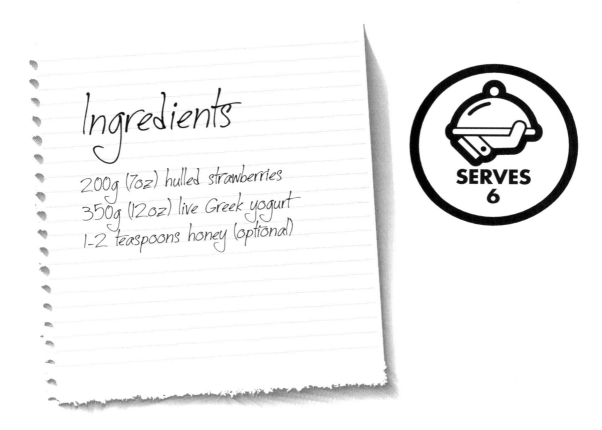

Ingredients

200g (7oz) hulled strawberries
350g (12oz) live Greek yogurt
1-2 teaspoons honey (optional)

SERVES
6

Method

Take around 6 medium strawberries and roughly chop them. Place the remaining strawberries, yogurt and honey (if using) into a food processor and whizz until smooth and creamy. Spoon some of the yogurt mixture into lolly moulds only filling each one about half way. Pop a few pieces of chopped strawberry into each mould then continue to spoon the remaining mixture in. Press the remaining strawberry pieces into the moulds. Place them into the freezer for around 2 hours or until they have completely set. Ready to eat whenever you are ready.

Baked Peach Melba

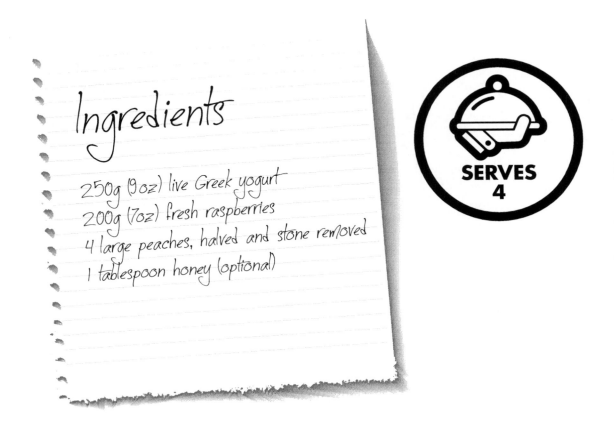

Ingredients

250g (9oz) live Greek yogurt
200g (7oz) fresh raspberries
4 large peaches, halved and stone removed
1 tablespoon honey (optional)

SERVES
4

Method

Place the peach halves onto a baking tray and drizzle a little honey (if using) over the top. Bake them in the oven at 180C/360F for 10 minutes. In the meantime, place the raspberries into a food processor and blitz until smooth. Serve the peach halves onto plates with a dollop of yogurt on the side. Drizzle the raspberry sauce over the top. Eat straight away.

HOMEMADE PROBIOTICS

Sauerkraut

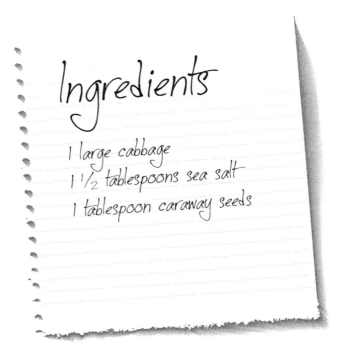

Ingredients

1 large cabbage
1 ½ tablespoons sea salt
1 tablespoon caraway seeds

Method

Chop the cabbage very finely. You may want to use a food processor for this. Make sure all your equipment is sterile. Place the chopped cabbage in a large bowl and add in the caraway seeds and salt. Using clean hands massage the salt and caraway seeds into the cabbage and let it stand for 10 minutes or so. Using glass jars or food containers, spoon the mixture into them, pressing it down so that the cabbage is completely submerged in the brine. This enable fermentation to take place.

Cover the containers with a paper towel and place an elastic band around the neck to form a lid. This will protect it but still let the air in. Store in a cool place. Check daily that the cabbage is covered and press it down if you need to. Remove any scum as it develops and bubbles appearing are a good sign that it is fermenting. As a guide, the sauerkraut can be fermented after 3 days but more likely it can take 2 weeks to a month. You can always taste it as it develops. After one month it should be done enough and can be kept in the fridge in an airtight container.

Kefir

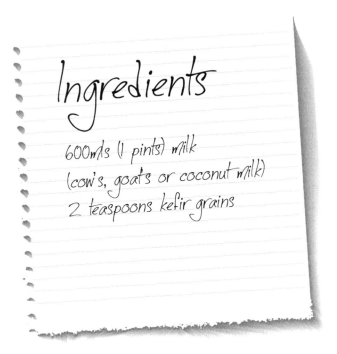

Ingredients

600mls (1 pints) milk
(cow's, goats or coconut milk)
2 teaspoons kefir grains

Method

If you have bought dried kefir grains you will need to activate them. You can do this by soaking them in milk (full-fat) for 3-6 days, changing the milk daily.

Place the milk and kefir grains in a glass jar or container and stir. Cover the container with a paper towel, secured with an elastic band to form a breathable lid. Keep the container at room temperature for 24 hours. If it is tangy to taste and has thickened it is ready to drink although it may take up to 48 hours to ferment properly. Strain the mixture to sieve out the kefir grains and it is ready to drink. Keep the grains to use on another batch and repeat the process. If you don't want another batch of kefir straight away you can store them in milk in the fridge ready to reuse. Never use a screw top lid as this can create a vacuum and may be dangerous with a glass jar.

Kimchi

Ingredients

- 6 large radishes, grated (shredded)
- 5 spring onions (scallions) finely chopped
- 2 large carrots, grated (shredded)
- 1 Chinese leaf cabbage, finely chopped, washed and dried
- 4 cloves of garlic, finely chopped
- 2.5cm (1inch) chunk of fresh ginger, finely chopped
- 1 1/2-2 tablespoons chilli sauce
- 1 tablespoon sea salt
- 3 tablespoons rice vinegar

Method

In a bowl, combine the radishes, onions, carrots, ginger, salt, garlic, chilli and vinegar and mix well. Place the cabbage into a large bowl and stir in the salt. Set it aside for 30 minutes. Add the chilli mixture to the cabbage and mix well. Spoon the mixture into thoroughly cleaned glass jars or food containers. Press the mixture down well so that the vegetables are completely submerged. Cover them with a paper towel secured with an elastic band to create a breathable lid. Leave it to ferment overnight then keep it in the fridge until ready to use.

Yogurt

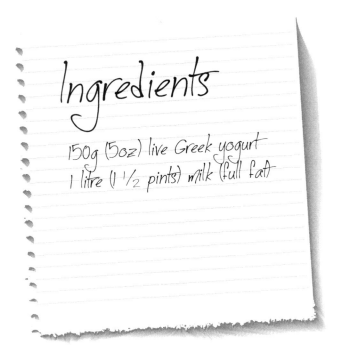

Ingredients

150g (5oz) live Greek yogurt
1 litre (1 ½ pints) milk (full fat)

Method

Pour the milk into a large saucepan and warm it to 40C (you'll need a thermometer for this). Remove the milk from the heat. Stir in the live yogurt and mix it really well. It's the cultures in the live yogurt that transform the milk into yogurt. Transfer the yogurt to a large bowl or if you have a yogurt maker pour it into that. Cover the bowl with a clean tea towel and let it stand at room temperature for 7-8 hours. Spoon the mixture into a glass jars or a lidded container and store in the fridge until ready to eat. It's essential the yogurt you use for this is live.

You may also be interested in other titles by
Erin Rose Publishing
which are available in both paperback and ebook.

 Quick Start Guides

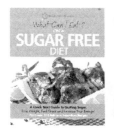 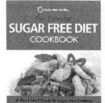 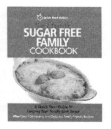 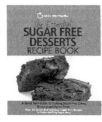 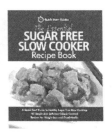

    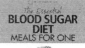

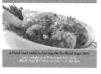 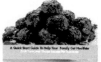

  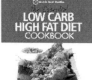 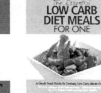 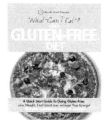

 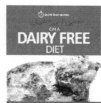 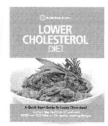 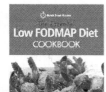

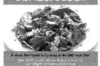

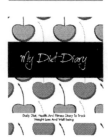 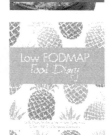 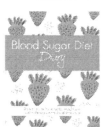 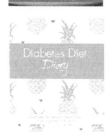 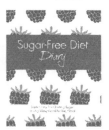

Books by Sophie Ryan
Erin Rose Publishing

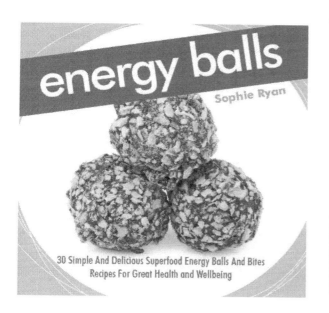

30 Simple And Delicious Superfood Energy Balls And Bites
Recipes For Great Health and Wellbeing

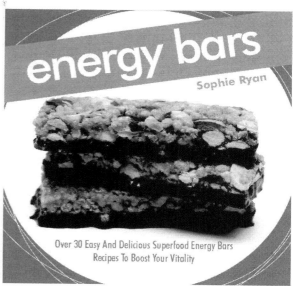

Over 30 Easy And Delicious Superfood Energy Bars
Recipes To Boost Your Vitality

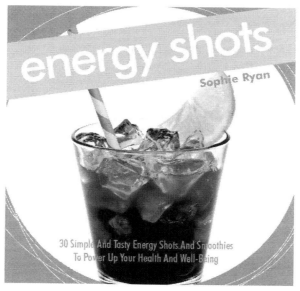

30 Simple And Tasty Energy Shots And Smoothies
To Power Up Your Health And Well-Being

Printed in Great Britain
by Amazon

16927204R00070